Heart Defects
in Children
What Every Parent Should Know

Dedicated with love to my son, Stephen H. Wild.

Mommy loves you!

Heaven's Very Special Child

A meeting was held quite far from Earth!
It's time again for another birth.
Said the Angels to the Lord above,
This Special Child will need much Love.
His progress may be very slow,
Accomplishment he may not show.
And he'll need extra care,
From the folks he meets down there.
He may not run or laugh or play,
His thoughts may seem quite far away.
In many ways he won't adapt,
And he'll be known as handicapped.
So let's be careful where he's sent.
We want his life to be content.
Please Lord, find the parents who,
Will do a special job for you.
They will not realize right away,
The leading role they're asked to play.
But with this child sent from above,
Comes stronger faith, and richer Love.
And soon they'll know the privilege given,
In caring for their gift from Heaven.
Their precious charge so meek and mild,
Is Heaven's Very Special Child.

—Author Unknown

Heart Defects in Children
What Every Parent Should Know

Cheryl J. Wild
R.N., B.S.N.
Adult, Pediatric, and Neonatal
Surgical Intensive Care Nurse
Open Heart Surgery

Medical Editor
Michael J. Neary, MD
Director of the Surgical Open
Heart Intensive Care Unit
Deborah Heart and Lung Center
Browns Mills, New Jersey

CHRONIMED PUBLISHING

Heart Defects in Children: What Every Parent Should Know
© 1999 by Cheryl Wild, R.N., B.S.N.

Library of Congress Cataloging-in-Publication Data
Wild, Cheryl
Heart defects in children / by Cheryl Wild

     p.   cm.

Includes index.

ISBN 1-56561-166-7

Acquiring Editor: Cheryl Kimball
Copy Editor: Renée Nicholls
Text Design & Production: David Enyeart
Art/Production Manager: Claire Lewis
Illustrations: Pat Rouse
Cover Design: Pear Graphic Design

Printed in the United States

Published by
Chronimed Publishing
P.O. Box 59032
Minneapolis, MN 55459-0032

10   9   8   7   6   5   4   3   2   1

Notice: Consult a Health Care Professional. Because individual cases and needs vary, readers are advised to seek the guidance of a licensed physician, registered dietitian, or other health care professional before making changes in their health care regimen. This book is intended for informational purposes only and is not for use as an alternative to appropriate medical care. While every effort has been made to ensure that the information is the most current available, new research findings, being released with increasing frequency, may invalidate some data.

I believe this work to be one of those uncommon little books that truly fulfill a need. In this case, it is an explanatory text for concerned parents of very special patients, those with congenital heart disease. It serves to clarify wonderfully a topic that can be very complex for anyone, medical and layperson alike. It was prepared with a great deal of love and respect. It will be read, I believe, with an equal measure of both ingredients.

—Dr. Michael J. Neary, Director
Surgical Intensive Care Unit
Deborah Heart and Lung Center

Contents

Part Four—Personalizing Your Child's Defect and Repair with the Use of Draw-On Hearts

Appendices

Preface

I have been a nurse for ten years, and I have been a mother for five. The day my son Stephen was born was the most incredible, amazing day of my life. My pregnancy was a hard one. My placenta had partially ruptured off of the uterine wall when I was about six and a half months along. Doctor after doctor could not stop the contractions that I had as a result of the tearing. My baby's lungs were not mature enough to support him yet, and he would have to fight for life on a ventilator if he was born too early. I was very frightened, and was admitted into a "high risk" city hospital for the remainder of my pregnancy. Thank God, we did OK. During my hospitalization, I had the pleasure of meeting many new parents. Because of the high-risk stature of the hospital nursery, a lot of them were suffering because their new babies were born with congenital heart defects.

Finally, I felt that I could be of use. My training and specialty as a nurse was in cardiac care. I had been working for the previous six years in a surgical intensive care unit taking care of adults and children of all ages after heart surgery. From my hospital bed, I began to teach. Many of the babies were premature, and most of the heart defects I encountered were common ones. I would get as much information from the parents as I could, and try to explain to them how serious or not serious their child's particular defect was.

I realized through these experiences that in times of stress, parents cannot retain specific information that is thrown at them by the medical staff. Even if the information they received was positive, these moms and dads only really heard the scary stuff. I did the same thing. The closer I got to delivering, the more frightened I

9

became, and the less I really heard what the doctors were saying. It was then that I realized I could really help the parents of these children—in writing.

I did some research, and I found that there are many medical journals and textbooks that explain children's congenital heart defects to doctors, medical students, and nurses. But it is the parents who so often need to know the what, where, why, and how. So I have, to the best of my ability, simplified the "medical jargon." It is here in black and white, so that your questions may be answered again and again, in terms that are easier to understand than a rambling physician, on a stressful day.

I have included the most common defects that you will be exposed to. There are, however, other defects that may not be mentioned here. If you need written explanations of a defect not covered in this book, please speak directly with your medical support team. Ask them to explain the anatomy, draw pictures, and provide you with explanations of the symptoms your child may experience. In addition, have them write down any treatment options you may have, medical and surgical, and ask them to explain exactly what expectations you and your child should have for the future.

My hope is that I can help parents understand. With education and understanding, we will all be better able to cope successfully with the daily life that affects each child with a congenital heart defect.

Medical technology is advancing, and our physicians are becoming more and more skilled in the treatment of congenital heart defects. We are therefore seeing an increase in the survival rates, and most important, the quality of life for the children.

This book is for the children.

Acknowledgments

With many thanks to my mother, Patricia Belz, a lady with re-markable strength and courage. And, to my father, John Hansen, who taught me that "what we do, and what we say, makes us who we are." To my aunt Dorothy Brodka, through her love I learned parenting, patience, and kindness. To Thomas, Robert, John, and Bryan, my Hansen brothers, who taught me love and helped me to believe in myself. (Also to my sister-in-law, Kerri, and my brother-in-law, Luke, who chose to belong to this rat pack.) Thanks to my best friend and confidant, Cheryl Falcey Gray, who was with me at the inception of this book. She followed through many difficult times with me, and never offered anything less than praise and encouragement. To Dr. Michael J. Neary for being my advisor and sounding board during difficult times, and his right arm, Theresa Young. Thank you Maria Fiorinelli for making Oliver a home. Thank you Jeffrey Ojaniit for teaching me strength and reminding me how important it is to love. We grow only when we push our-selves beyond what we already know. To Eric Smith for restoring my faith in the "happily ever after." I love you, and I believe in us. And finally, to my friends and colleagues in the Pediatric Surgical In-tensive Care Unit at Deborah Heart and Lung Center. They are among the most skilled and talented group of professionals I have ever had the pleasure of working with. Keep the faith, and remember what awesome feats you accomplish every day.

How to Use This Book

In the beginning chapters of this book, you will learn how a healthy heart functions, and what changes take place in a baby's heart when it is born. After you have read Part One, move ahead to Part Two and choose the chapter that best describes your child's personal heart defect. If that defect is not listed in Chapters 4 through 10, use the outline for heart defects in Chapter 11 and have your doctors help you create your own personal guide. When you are finished reading about your child's defect, move ahead again to Chapter 12 and read through the rest of the book. Do not hesitate to make notations in the book, and write down any questions you may have that can be answered by your physicians.

The information on each heart defect is general. It is important for you to know that any two children who appear to have the same defect will not be exactly the same, so don't compare your child to another. Please feel free to use the "Draw-On Hearts" at the back of this book to personalize your child's defect and repair.

Part One
The Heart

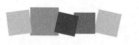

CHAPTER I

Introduction to and Causes of Heart Defects

Congenital Heart Defects

It is estimated that one in every one hundred babies born today has a congenital heart defect. About one-third of these children are considered to be in critical condition. A large number of these very sick, "critical" babies used to die before they reached the age of one (one-third in the first week of their lives). Today however, 60 percent of the critical children live well past their first year, and some will even go on to lead full healthy lives. We can attribute this to expanding knowledge and advancing medical technology.

"Congenital heart defect," is a phrase that the medical field uses to group a large number of heart conditions in children. Basically, it means that your child was born with a defect, or an abnormality, in the structure of the heart. It may be the persistence of fetal circulation after birth, or it may be from malformation (misdevelopment of the heart as it is forming in utero).

Persistent Fetal Circulation

A baby's heart goes through many changes as the baby adjusts to life outside its mother's body. The fetal heart works differently and has many different characteristics than the newborn baby's heart. At birth, there are structural changes that take place in the heart. These changes are the result of pressure fluctuations in the atmosphere, from life in the uterus (which may be like living underwater), to independent life on earth. Fetal circulation can persist after birth if the changes that should occur at birth do not. Babies that are born prematurely have a higher incidence of defects caused by persistent fetal circulation.

Some defects caused by the persistence of fetal circulation will correct themselves spontaneously with time. Still other defects may need the assistance of medicine and/or surgery. The most common heart defects caused by persistent fetal circulation are Atrial Septal Defects (ASDs), and Patent Ductus Arteriosis (PDAs). Refer to Chapters 4 and 5 for a more detailed explanation of these defects.

Misdevelopment

There are many causes for the misdevelopment of a baby's heart as it is forming within the womb. Your genes and your environment can influence the development of a child in utero, but it is rarely easy to pinpoint the direct cause of most defects.

Years ago, researchers were able to directly link certain birth defects with the ingestion or exposure to a teratogen. A *teratogen* is anything that can cause a deformity, or an unnatural development, in unborn babies. If a mother is exposed to a certain drug, chemical, or disease during pregnancy, harmful effects may result to her baby's development. Scientists were able to show a relationship between the use of certain medications such as Thalidomide and Dilantin and the occurrence of certain birth defects. Similarly, the excessive use of alcohol by a mother during pregnancy has been linked to birth defects. Also found to be culprits were some viruses, including rubella, which causes measles-type symptoms in children but is very harmful to a developing fetus. These teratogens are especially dangerous if the mother is exposed to them during the early stages of her baby's heart development, in her first trimester. Teratogens, however, really only account for a very small portion of heart defects.

Sometimes a congenital heart defect can be attributed to your genetic makeup. A person's genetic makeup is handed down from generation to generation. If a person has two or more family members previously affected with a congenital heart defect, that person has a "strong family history." In this case, the gene causing a specific defect might be passed on from the parent to the child. If your child has been born with a defect, and your family history for congenital heart defects is strong, your doctor might recommend genetic counseling before you consider having more children.

Other genetic causes of heart defects involve children who are born with chromosomal abnormalities such as Down's syndrome or Turner's syndrome. These conditions are characterized by varying

Heart Defects in Children

degrees of mental retardation and multiple developmental defects. Heart defects have been found in approximately 40 percent of patients with Down's syndrome, and among 20 to 40 percent of patients with Turner's syndrome. There are special books available for parents whose children may be afflicted with these chromosomal conditions. The heart defects most commonly associated with these syndromes can be found in the chapters that follow.

It is very important for you to know that most children who are born with a heart defect have no family history and no risk factors at all! It is not known why these defects occur, and there is absolutely no one to blame. As parents, we always try to find the "how" and the "why." In most cases it is important for us to let go of this and move on to the "what now"—playing the hand we have been dealt in order to meet the needs of our very special child.

Most experts will agree that if there is no family history, there is no reason to believe that any other children born to the same parents will be affected with a heart defect. The low recurrence rate in additional births and the increasing possibilities for treatment will usually justify having more children.

In the chapters that follow, you will learn new things, find answers to at least some of your present questions, and hopefully generate many new questions. The information on each defect is *general.* No two children with the same defect will act and react the same way to the defect or to the treatment. Compile for yourself a list of any and all questions you may have, as they enter your mind. If they are unanswered throughout this book, be sure to approach your medical support team with them. Remember, the doctors, nurses, and therapists are working for you!

CHAPTER 2

The Healthy Heart

TO PROPERLY UNDERSTAND how a heart with a defect works, it is first important to understand how a normal heart works. This chapter will help you visualize how blood makes its way through the body.

The Circulatory System

The circulatory system is made up of blood, arteries, capillaries, veins, and the heart.

Blood

Think of blood as a liquid that consists of many different types of cells with varying functions. Its major jobs are to transport oxygen and nutrients around the body, and to carry off waste products such as carbon dioxide. Blood makes a complete circle around the body in approximately twenty seconds!

Arteries

All arteries carry blood away from the heart (a good way to remember this is "A for Away"). Arteries carry oxygenated, or fresh, blood, which is high in nutrients and is used to fuel the body. (The exception is the pulmonary artery, which carries deoxygenated blood to the lungs.) Arteries bring this freshly oxygenated blood to all of the organs and tissues of our bodies.

Capillaries

Capillaries are tiny blood vessels between arteries and veins. They act like filters. When blood reaches the end of an artery, it slowly

FIGURE 2-1
THE CIRCULATORY SYSTEM

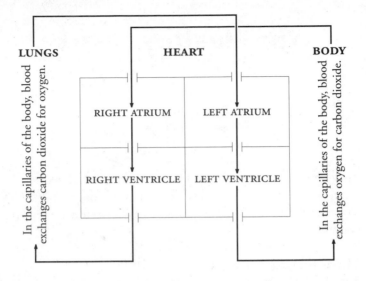

squeezes through the capillaries. As it does, oxygen is filtered out through the capillary walls and enters the surrounding tissues. Our tissues use the oxygen and other nutrients as energy so the muscles can work efficiently. When oxygen is used in our body, carbon dioxide and waste products are produced. The carbon dioxide and the waste products leak back through the capillary walls, and the blood carries it off through the veins.

Veins

Veins carry deoxygenated, or "used," blood from the body to the heart. (The exception is the pulmonary vein, which returns oxygenated blood from the lungs to the heart.) You may have heard this blood referred to as "blue blood." The veins that you see on the back of your hand are themselves blue, but the blood in those veins is always red. The color blue can appear in your body if the oxygen content in your tissues is low. Veins carry deoxygenated blood. But if you cut a vein, the blood itself is red.

Sometimes your skin can look blue. Children with a congenital heart defect can have bluish skin, called *cyanosis,* if the oxygen content in their blood is low. But you do not have to be sick to have blue skin. If you are cold, your tissues will constrict to preserve heat. When the tissues constrict, pressure around the capillaries makes it difficult for the oxygenated blood to leak out into the surrounding tissue. The tissues become low in oxygen and will appear as bluish nails or lips—just as children get blue lips if they are in a cold pool of water.

The Heart

The heart is a large muscle with four hollow chambers. It lies behind your breastbone and tilts to the left side of your chest. It is protected by the ribs and by various layers of muscles and tissues. The four chambers consist of two atria and two ventricles. The atria are on the top, one to the left and one to the right; the ventricles sit below them. The function of the heart is to circulate blood throughout the body. It does this by collecting, passing, and pumping blood. The atria collect blood and pass it through the valves of the heart to the ventricles. The ventricles pump the blood out of the heart and around the body.

THE RIGHT SIDE OF THE HEART The function of the right side of the heart (Figure 2-2, next page) is to gather used blood from the body and circulate it to the lungs, where it can be reoxygenated. All deoxygenated (used) blood from the body returns to the right side of the heart through two large veins called the superior and inferior vena cavas. These veins carry blood from all parts of the body and empty it into the right atrium, where the blood collects. When the atrium is full, it contracts, and the blood is forced to pass through a valve called the tricuspid valve. This valve allows the blood to flow down into the right ventricle.

Once the right ventricle is filled with deoxygenated blood from the right atrium, it forcefully contracts. Blood is pumped through the pulmonary valve, and into the pulmonary artery toward the lungs. In the capillaries of the lungs, the oxygen we have breathed in enters the blood stream, and carbon dioxide is exhaled. (If you are a smoker, beware—the air that you have breathed in may be inadequate to maintain healthy tissues.) The newly oxygenated blood is circulated out of the lungs, through the pulmonary veins, and the left side of the heart takes over.

FIGURE 2-2
THE HEALTHY HEART

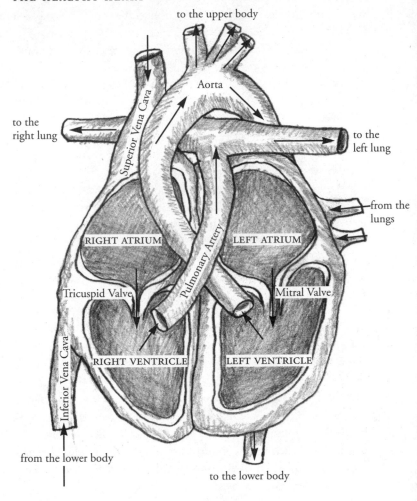

to the upper body

Aorta

Superior Vena Cava

to the
right lung

to the
left lung

from the
lungs

RIGHT ATRIUM

LEFT ATRIUM

Pulmonary Artery

Tricuspid Valve

Mitral Valve

Inferior Vena Cava

RIGHT VENTRICLE

LEFT VENTRICLE

from the lower body

to the lower body

THE LEFT SIDE OF THE HEART The left side of the heart (see
Figure 2-2) has the most important job of all. Its responsibility is to
gather blood from the lungs and forcefully pump it to the body.
The left atrium collects the freshly oxygenated blood from the pulmonary veins (coming from the lungs). When the atrium is full it
contracts, and the blood is passed through the mitral valve into the
left ventricle. The left ventricle is the workhorse of the heart. It gen-

erates very high pressures with its muscular pumping, and blood is ejected through the aortic valve into the aorta. The aorta is the largest artery in the body. Blood is sent from the heart through the aorta to all of the arteries and tissues in the body.

The pressure generated by the left ventricle is well known as "blood pressure." A normal blood pressure in a healthy young adult is approximately 120/70. These numbers indicate how hard the left ventricle must work to effectively pump blood around your body. The higher the numbers are, the harder the heart is working. When you feel a pulse in your wrist, you are actually feeling your arteries vibrate with the blood flow.

HOW THE SIDES WORK TOGETHER Although it may sound like the two sides of the heart are separate, they actually work together very efficiently. The atria both contract together, pushing blood simultaneously through the tricuspid valve (on the right side) and the mitral valve (on the left side). Then, the ventricles contract together, pushing blood through the pulmonic valve (on the right side) and the aortic valve (on the left side). Deoxygenated blood enters the lungs for gas exchange from the right side. At the same time, oxygenated blood enters the body to fuel our tissues from the left side. Imagine, one red blood cell can circulate the body in approximately twenty seconds. The blood cell gets pumped out of the left ventricle, bringing fuel to the body, and comes back through the veins to the right atrium. The right ventricle sends the blood cell back out of the heart to the lungs, where it gets reoxygenated. After the blood cell is done in the lungs, it returns again to the left atrium, where it begins its journey all over. This completes the "circle" of the circulatory system.

Murmurs

The large pumping chambers in the heart (the ventricles) force the valves to open and close. When the valves close, they cause the "lub-dub" sounds of your heartbeat. When doctors listen to your heart, they can tell many different things about blood flow, and especially about the condition of the valves. Certain diseases, defects, or infections can cause changes in the shapes of the valves. When the damaged valves close, the closure may be incomplete and some blood may leak back through the valve (this is called *regurgitation*). When this happens, an abnormal sound called a *murmur* can be heard. The seriousness of the murmur will depend on the amount of damage there is at the valve.

Murmurs can also be heard if there are defects in the structure of the heart and its vessels, or if there is persistence of fetal circulation. In these cases, a murmur would mean that there was abnormal shunting (diverting) of blood across a membrane that should normally be intact, or through a passageway that should be closed. Doctors can become proficient in diagnosing these sounds depending on where they put their stethoscopes on your chest to listen.

If your child is diagnosed as having a heart murmur, don't fret. Something called an *innocent murmur* happens in approximately 50 percent of all children. Innocent murmurs occur without defects, or abnormalities, in the heart. Innocent murmurs, however, should never be accompanied by cyanosis (bluish skin) or any other symptoms. I always recommended follow-up diagnostic tests to confirm the cause of any murmur found in a child. As always, speak directly—and without hesitation—to your physicians regarding your child's health.

CHAPTER 3

Before Your Baby Was Born

CIRCULATION IN AN unborn child's heart is difficult to understand. Review this chapter slowly and refer frequently to the pictures. Try to visualize the path that blood takes in the fetal heart.

Approximately two weeks after mom's egg is fertilized, the fetal heart will begin to develop. Although it is beating by the twenty-fourth day, it does not look like a heart. At first, it resembles a long hollow tube, but it slowly changes, by twisting and out-patching, into a four-chambered muscular pump. By the forty-fifth day, the heart is fully developed, but it will continue to grow and mature until well after the child is born.

Every artery and vein that is attached to the heart is positioned very carefully. Each vessel has a specific job for the direction of blood flow through it. With every contraction of the heart, an artery sends blood to a certain organ, tissue, or cell within the body. If there is any disruption in the formation of the heart or its vessels during development, such as a congenital heart defect, blood flow through the body can be altered.

The unborn baby is dramatically different from a newborn child. Unlike a newborn, a fetus will get all of its nutrients from mom's placenta. The placenta is an organ that is attached to the inside wall of the mother's uterus. An umbilical cord comes from the placenta and enters the fetus through its belly button. Through this cord, mom can supply all of the baby's nutritional needs. If the placenta is not functional, the fetus cannot survive.

A fetus does not breathe air. Its lungs are deflated and they are filled with fluid. All of the oxygen it needs comes from mom's placenta. Because the lungs are not functional, blood does not need to

FIGURE 3-1

CIRCULATION IN THE FETAL HEART

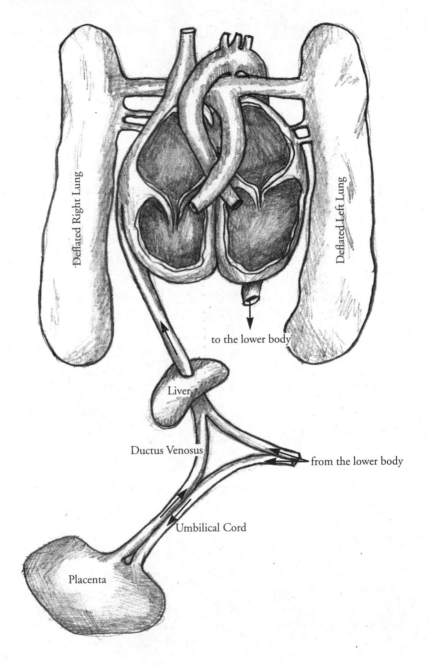

Deflated Right Lung

Deflated Left Lung

to the lower body

Liver

Ductus Venosus

from the lower body

Umbilical Cord

Placenta

flow to them for oxygen. Therefore, the fetal body develops a way to shunt (divert) blood away from the lungs (where it does not need to go), and toward the developing body, where it is needed more. Because of this shunting of the blood flow, only about 8 to 10 percent of the blood that is in the heart will go to the lungs. (All blood flow in a newborn baby's heart goes to the lungs.) Blood that does enter a fetus's lungs will circulate out (not oxygenated) and return to the left side of the heart (the left atrium), just as blood in the newborn's heart would.

There are three ways that blood is shunted in a fetal heart. They are temporary for the fetus, and are disassembled during birth. These shunts are difficult to understand. Their technical names are:

• the ductus venosus;
• the foramen ovale; and
• the ductus arteriosus.

For help with the following paragraphs, please refer frequently to the diagrams provided.

The Ductus Venosus

Because the fetal lungs do not have air in them, the fetus must get oxygen from mom's placenta. The ductus venosus (Figure 3–1) is a vein in the umbilical cord that enters through the belly button. It carries all of the nutrients and oxygen that a developing fetus will need to survive. This vein creates a special channel through the baby's abdomen, and attaches to a large vein (the inferior vena cava) that enters the heart directly. This allows blood from the placenta to gain direct access into the fetal heart. The heart pumps this new blood to the body, where it can then be utilized for growth and energy.

The Foramen Ovale

The foramen ovale (Figure 3–2) is an opening in the wall of the fetal heart that separates the two upper chambers. It looks like a hole between the right and left atria. In a newborn child, the right and left sides of the heart are separate, and blood cannot mix between them. But the fetal heart is different. Blood does not need to travel through the right side of the heart at all. Once a child is born, the right side of the heart sends blood to the lungs for oxygen, but the fetus gets all of its oxygen from mom's placenta, and its lungs are deflated. It only needs 8 to 10 percent of the blood flow from its heart.

This foramen ovale shunts approximately 40 percent of the blood that enters the heart through the right atrium (from mom's placenta and its little body) across to the left atrium. It completely bypasses the lungs. Once the blood is in the left atrium, it can pass through the mitral valve and be pumped by the left ventricle directly to the body.

Because the foramen ovale shunts almost half of the blood from the right atrium to the left, the right ventricle and the pulmonary artery do not get a lot of blood. In fact, the right ventricle and the pulmonary artery only have to work at about one half of their potential before the child is born. Once the child is born, the foramen ovale will close. At that time, the right ventricle and the pulmonary artery will have to accommodate 100 percent of the blood flow through the heart. If there is a defect in the baby's right ventricle, pulmonary artery, or lungs, it may not be noticed until after the baby is born, when the shunts close and these areas of the heart receive 100 percent of the blood flow. Until then, they may be virtually undetectable.

FIGURE 3-2

THE FORAMEN OVALE

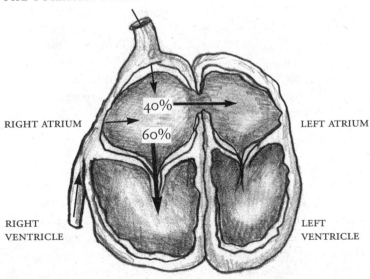

RIGHT ATRIUM   40%   LEFT ATRIUM

60%

RIGHT VENTRICLE   LEFT VENTRICLE

FIGURE 3-3
THE DUCTUS ARTERIOSUS

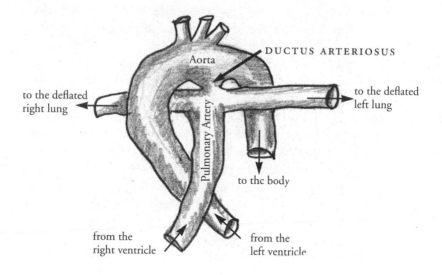

The Ductus Arteriosus

The ductus arteriosus (Figure 3-3) looks like a small straw. It connects the pulmonary artery, which brings blood to the lungs, to the aorta, which sends blood to the body. Because of the foramen ovale, only about 60 percent of the blood in the right atrium, will make it down into the right ventricle. The blood that does make it is pumped into the pulmonary artery toward the nonfunctioning lungs. Remember, blood does not need to flow to the lungs because mom is supplying all of the oxygen through the placenta. The purpose of the ductus arteriosus is to shunt that blood away from the fetal lungs. Most of the blood that enters the pulmonary artery (approximately 90 percent) is diverted through the ductus arteriosus directly into the aorta. This blood completely bypasses the lungs and is sent straight to the body, where it is needed for energy. Only about 10 percent of blood will get by this shunt and flow to the lungs, not for oxygen but to give the lung tissues energy to grow too.

In a newborn, all blood in the aorta has been pumped there from the left ventricle. But in the fetus, most of the blood never had to be pumped by the left ventricle. It was shunted to the aorta through the ductus arteriosus. So before birth, the left ventricle only works at about one third of its potential. After the child is born, the ductus arteriosus will close, and the left ventricle will have to pump 100 percent of the blood flow. This is why if there are any defects or problems with the left ventricle or the aorta, they may be virtually undetectable until after birth.

Sometimes, two of the shunts, the ductus arteriosus and the foramen ovale, will remain open (patent) after birth, and blood will continue to shunt through them. There are many reasons why these shunts do not close. If there is a defect present in the heart, the shunts may remain functioning to assist the flow of blood through the heart and to the body. In this case, a patent ductus arteriosus and foramen ovale that remains open after birth may be beneficial to the heart. Measures can be taken to keep them open and functioning until the defect is corrected so proper blood flow can be restored for the child. But the ductus arteriosus and foramen ovale may also continue shunting blood for other reasons that doctors cannot explain. This condition is simply called "Persistent Fetal Circulation." It can be common in babies who are born prematurely. These shunts may eventually close by themselves, but sometimes they will need medical or surgical assistance.

Unlike a newborn, a fetus does not have arteries that are high in oxygen. Its blood is relatively low in oxygen because the lungs don't function (remember, the blood is mixed in mom's placenta). The oxygen "saturation" (a measured percentage of oxygen in blood) is between 50 to 60 percent. A healthy newborn baby has an oxygen saturation of approximately 98 percent. This difference is why many newborns look blue when they are born. As they make the transition to independent life, their fetal shunts close, their lungs expand, they oxygenate themselves, and they become "pink."

The Miraculous Birth of a Baby

When a baby is born, major changes take place in its heart and lungs. There is a change in the atmospheric pressure around the lungs during birth, which will cause the baby to cry and breathe air. Some of the fluid that once filled the lungs is suctioned out of the nose by the medical staff, and the rest pushed into the capillaries by the air the baby breathes in. The fluid in the capillaries enters the veins, and becomes part of the blood stream. As this happens, more

Heart Defects in Children

pressure changes in the heart and lungs trigger the body to disassemble the two remaining fetal shunts.

Closing of the fetal shunts should occur naturally and will generally be completed within the first few days of the baby's life, to allow blood flow to get to the lungs for oxygen exchange. The ductus arteriosus, which connects the pulmonary artery to the aorta, will constrict and seal off. Blood in the pulmonary artery will now flow directly to the lungs to get oxygen for circulation in the body. The foramen ovale, on the wall between the atria, will flap closed because of the pressure changes between the two chambers. This "flap" closure of the shunt will close the hole, but may not permanently seal until the first few months of the baby's life. This closure will prevent blood from mixing between the right and left sides of the heart. Once these shunts are disassembled, the heart will have made the healthy transition between fetus and newborn.

Part Two
Your Child's Defect

CHAPTER 4

Atrial Septal Defects (ASDs)

AN ATRIAL SEPTAL DEFECT is commonly referred to as a "hole in the heart." More specifically, as its name explains, it is a defect, or opening, in the atrial septum (Figure 4–1, next page), which is the wall that separates the right and left atria. As we discussed in Chapter 2, the atria are the two smaller chambers on the top part of the heart. Their function is to collect blood from various parts of the body and pass it down through the valves to the ventricles. Although the atrial septum is normally open in the fetal heart (the foramen ovale), it should be closed in the child's heart. If it is not, abnormal mixing of right- and left-sided blood will occur.

Because all blood eventually goes through the entire body, you may wonder why mixing is considered bad. Remember that the blood in the right side of your heart is from the body, and it is headed for the lungs to be oxygenated. But blood in the left side of the heart is from the lungs, fresh with oxygen and headed toward the body for energy.

It really should not matter if a little fresh blood from the left atrium gets into the deoxygenated blood in the right atrium. That blood is going to the lungs anyway. But, problems may arise if there is a lot of mixing, and a lot of extra blood goes to the lungs. The baby's small pulmonary artery and tiny lungs may not be able to accommodate the extra blood flow.

If deoxygenated blood from the right side mixes across into the left side of the heart (where there is freshly oxygenated blood), the percentage of oxygen in the blood going to the body can be lowered. If it is only lowered a little, nothing bad may happen. But, if there is a lot of blood mixing from the right side into the left, there

FIGURE 4-1
ATRIAL SEPTAL DEFECT

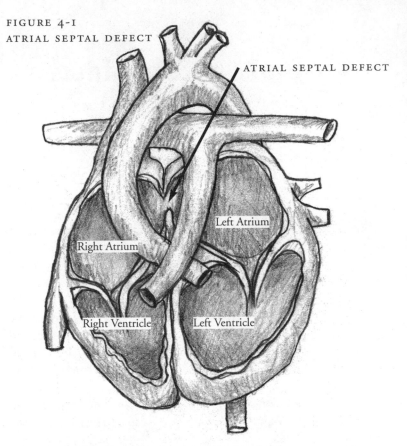

ATRIAL SEPTAL DEFECT

Left Atrium

Right Atrium

Right Ventricle

Left Ventricle

may not be enough oxygen circulating in the bloodstream to maintain pink tissues. This can be bad.

Luckily, the right and left atria contract at the same time, and the force of the contractions is pretty equal. This means that even if there is a defect in the wall that separates the atria (the atrial septum), there should not be a large amount of blood shunting back and forth unless the defect is very large, or if the septum itself is absent. In these cases, a lot of mixing of right- and left-sided blood can occur.

Symptoms to Watch For
Commonly, a child with an ASD will not have any symptoms at all. In fact, this defect is likely to go undetected until your child's first preschool medical exam. This is mostly because the murmur created

by an ASD is not easy to hear, and the child may look very healthy for a period of years, even with an ASD. Still, a small percentage of infants, children, and many adults with ASDs will have symptoms such as shortness of breath, frequent respiratory infections, and/or swelling in their legs and abdomen. Other children may get tired faster during play, or when they exercise.

Complications an ASD Can Cause
Pulmonary Vascular Obstructive Disease

Despite the fact that the majority of children with ASDs have no symptoms, this does not mean that they will not develop complications. There are some symptoms that may occur, but more significant and life-threatening than these is a problem called "pulmonary vascular obstructive disease." This is a devastating condition that is known to develop in approximately 5 to 10 percent of patients (usually over the age of twenty) who have uncorrected ASDs. This condition is not reversible, and in most cases it is fatal within a few years of its onset. Because of this, it is very important to carefully consider the surgical repair of every atrial septal defect.

Treatment You Can Expect

There is no medicine that will fix an ASD, but doctors will prescribe medicine to treat the symptoms. Refer to pages 137 through 139 for an explanation and description of some commonly used medications. Today, there are two approaches to fixing an ASD: catheter closure or surgical repair.

The Catheter Closure of an ASD

Some children who have a small, single defect in the center of the atrial septum might be considered for closure with a "catheter procedure." This is also known in some hospitals as a "double umbrella procedure." Usually, this procedure is not done in the operating room, and the child does not need surgery. This is an obvious advantage. Unlike surgery, there is very little discomfort during recovery. This procedure has been used since approximately 1989 in some hospitals. But it is still considered "new" in others.

The child is given medication to sleep. Then, in a cardiac catheterization lab equipped with special x-ray equipment, a team of doctors, nurses, and technicians will pass a tiny catheter into the child's veins.

Remember, all veins carry blood to the right side of the heart. This catheter follows the blood flow, and enters the right atrium. The catheter has a piece of plastic that opens like an umbrella at the end of it. This device is coated with material that allows cells to grow on it. Carefully, the catheter is passed through the hole in the atrial septum, and the umbrella device is opened. Once it is open, the doctor will pull back on the catheter so that it touches the septum. A second umbrellalike device is inserted on the opposite side of the hole and pushed forward to flatten against the first. When the hole is sealed, the two umbrella devices are released, and the catheter is removed.

Within a matter of days, cells form on the open umbrellas, and tissue begins to grow. This tissue that the body makes forms a mesh around the umbrellas to help seal the septum. As the child's heart matures and grows, the cells on the septum grow too, and the defect stays sealed. If the procedure is successful, no further treatment is necessary. Rarely, one of the umbrellas may dislodge during insertion or shortly after. In this case, surgery may be needed to remove the umbrellas and repair the defect.

Unfortunately, a large number of children with ASDs are not candidates for the double umbrella procedure. This is mostly because of the location, number, and/or size of their defects. In this case, surgical repair of the ASD is indicated.

Surgical Correction of an ASD

In the operating room, under anesthesia, a child's ASD can be repaired. This is open heart surgery. After the child is asleep with medication, doctors will make an incision down the center of the chest so they can visualize the heart. Or, an incision can be made under the arm, on the left side of the body (this is called a *thoracotomy incision*). The doctor will use whichever approach he or she is most comfortable with. As parents, you may want to know where the scar will be—ask your doctor. The scar from a thoracotomy incision may be more cosmetically pleasing, especially in girls.

The procedure for closing an ASD is similar to mending. Some small holes can be sutured closed, just as you might sew a small tear in your clothes. Others, which may be larger or oddly shaped, may require a patch. There are different patches that can be used to correct the hole. Most commonly, a piece of tissue is taken from the pericardium, which is a protective, skinlike sac that covers the heart. Because it is part of the growing body, this piece of pericardium can be placed over the hole in the heart. Growing muscle fibers on the septum mesh with the patch, and allow it to grow with the child.

There are other kinds of patches that can be used to cover an ASD. Synthetic (man-made), patches are also used. These patches are made from a special sterile fabric, and they are sutured over the hole much like a knee patch on a pair of trousers. Growing muscle fibers in the heart will mesh with these sterile patches as part of the body's natural healing process. The heart's tissue helps seal the septum and provides a smooth surface where there once was a hole.

When a child has any procedure that involves closure of an ASD, antibiotics will be used to combat and prevent any infection that might occur. Sometimes, antibiotics are used before the procedure, and almost always after.

What You and Your Child Can Expect in the Future

Once the ASD is fixed, if there are no complications, you can expect your child to lead a full normal, healthy life without limitations. There are, however, risks associated with open heart surgery, which you should review with your doctor before the surgery occurs. In general, the risks of surgical correction of an ASD are very low, so you and your child can feel reassured about having the surgery.

A Special Note to Parents

If your child has an ASD at the site of the fetal shunt (the foramen ovale) and is not having symptoms, there is some merit in waiting until the child is more than one year of age before doing surgery. This is primarily to make sure that the defect will not close on its own. According to most medical literature, after the child reaches age three, more waiting is rarely justified. Extra time only allows the child more chance to develop complications. In general, the sooner the problem is corrected, the better it is for your child.

In cases where an ASD is not the only congenital heart defect, there might be a good reason to keep the ASD open and shunting blood. For example, with a defect such as Tricuspid Atresia, an ASD can be life-saving. Refer to the chapters on any other defects that may be involved with your child. As always, consult with your physicians regarding your child's unique situation.

Interesting Facts About ASDs

- An ASD is the fifth most common heart defect in children.
- ASDs occur two times more often in females than in males.
- Many hospitals are reporting the surgical correction of ASDs in the past few years, with no failures.

CHAPTER 5

Patent Ductus Arteriosus (PDAs)

AS WE DISCUSSED in Chapter 3, the ductus arteriosus is normal in a fetal heart. It is a tubelike connection between the pulmonary artery (which brings blood to the lungs) and the aorta (which brings blood to the body). All of the oxygen that your baby needed in utero came from the placenta. The lungs did not need to function, so the body shunted blood away from them. The blood that was going to the lungs was diverted through the ductus arteriosus into the aorta. Once it was in the aorta, the blood was sent to all areas of the body where it was needed for growth and energy.

Major changes take place when a child is born, which cause your baby to cry and breathe air. When this happens, the lungs expand and begin to work. The child's body must adapt to independent life by allowing blood to flow to the lungs. The ductus arteriosus must constrict and close off to allow all of the blood in the pulmonary artery to flow to the lungs. Then, oxygen in the lungs can be circulated into the bloodstream, and the child can oxygenate independently (instead of relying on mom's placenta).

The ductus arteriosus should constrict and close within the first few hours after birth. Once it is closed, all of the blood in the pulmonary artery can flow to the lungs for oxygen. If the ductus arteriosus does not close after birth, blood will continue to shunt through it. This is what is called a Patent Ductus Arteriosus (PDA). Although it is considered normal in a fetal heart, it is abnormal in a child's heart (Figure 5-1).

You might think that the PDA would cause the blood to continue to shunt from the pulmonary artery into the aorta. But now that the child has been born, the child's heart is generating very high

FIGURE 5-1
PATENT DUCTUS ARTERIOSUS

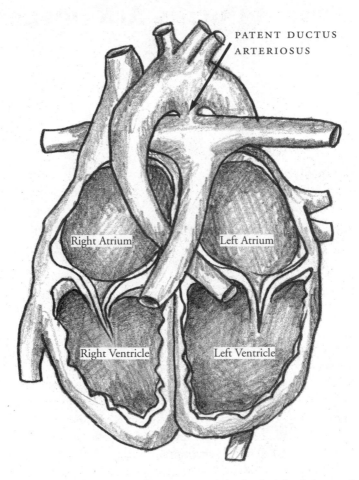

PATENT DUCTUS
ARTERIOSUS

Right Atrium

Left Atrium

Right Ventricle

Left Ventricle

pressure in order to pump blood around the body. The left ventricle is working very hard, and blood in the aorta is being forcefully ejected to the body. Consequently, the high-pressured blood in the aorta will eject down through the PDA and into the pulmonary artery. This is in the opposite direction from the blood flow in fetal circulation.

If blood is ejected from the aorta through the PDA, less oxygenated blood will get to your child's body for fuel and energy. What is more important, however, is the increased amount of blood going into the child's tiny pulmonary arteries and young lungs. If the PDA is large, a lot of blood will shunt through it, and the lungs may not be able to accommodate the increase in blood flow.

Symptoms to Watch For

Commonly, children with PDAs may not have any symptoms at all. If any symptoms do develop, they are proportional to the size of the PDA. The larger the shunt, the more symptoms occur. Some PDAs begin to constrict after birth, but they fail to close completely. The only symptom that these children may have is a heart murmur (extra sound) from the turbulent blood flow through the passageway. Some children may also have a small amount of cyanosis (blueness) of the lips and fingernails.

If the PDA is large and a lot of arterial blood shunts through it, more symptoms will appear. In extreme cases, symptoms of congestive heart failure may occur at a very young age (from infancy on). This condition is caused by circulatory congestion, or an overload of fluid, which makes the heart work extra hard. Such children may be short of breath or may breathe shallowly and rapidly. They may have swelling in the liver or abdomen, and they may grow slower than other children their age.

Complications a PDA Can Cause
Bacterial Endocarditis

If a PDA is left untreated, it can cause many problems. Bacterial endocarditis (see Chapter 12) is common in untreated patients. This is a very serious condition that involves infection and swelling in the heart and its valves. It is caused by many different forms of bacteria and can be treated with antibiotics. The chances of a child with a PDA developing Bacterial Endocarditis is estimated to be approximately 0.5 percent per year. These chances increase each year that the PDA is left open, but surgical correction of the defect will usually eliminate the risks of contracting this infection.

Pulmonary Vascular Disease

Another serious complication of a PDA is the onset of Pulmonary Vascular Disease. This condition is caused by years of abnormally increased blood flow to the lungs. The lungs respond by generating high pressures to keep the excess blood away. As a result, the body becomes stressed, and other complications arise. Pulmonary Vascular Disease is very serious, and it is not reversible. Because of these possible serious complications, every PDA should be treated.

Medical Treatment You Can Expect
Oxygen
To prevent the onset of complications, nearly every PDA should be closed. The way it can be closed depends mostly on your child's age and on the amount of blood being shunted through the defect. In a newborn infant, treatment with high levels of oxygen might help close the PDA. Premature infants, however, don't usually respond to oxygen in this way. And with a large majority of PDAs in newborns, oxygen does not work at all.

Medications
There is a medicine that will work with some children to close a PDA. This medicine is called Indomethacin (also known as Indocin). Exactly how Indocin works to close a PDA is not known. Doctors think that Indocin stops the body from making prostaglandins, which are strong hormones that, among other things, are known to work directly on the PDA to keep it open. Therefore, Indocin should block the effect of the prostaglandins and promote the natural closure of the PDA. Unfortunately, treatment with Indocin has only been found to affect the PDAs of premature infants. It seems to have less effect on babies who were born at full term. This means that unless Indocin is used immediately after a premature birth, it may not work. The trick is early detection, which is difficult because the child is not likely to have any symptoms. So, Indocin's power is limited.

Catheter Closures and Surgical Correction
If oxygen and medication fail to work, or your child has grown past the age of the effectiveness of these treatments, there are two approaches available today to correct a PDA: catheter closure, and surgical correction. Your child's age and size are rarely obstacles to surgery, even in the smallest of babies. Today, surgical correction of a PDA (in the operating room) is a proven form of treatment with minimal risk, minimal complications, and good results. A catheter closure procedure is also being performed in several hospitals throughout the country.

Heart Defects in Children

CATHETER CLOSURE OF A PDA Catheter closure of a PDA is currently limited to children over the age of eighteen months. This is mostly because the child's veins must be large enough to accommodate the catheters that are used in the procedure. The PDA must also be small enough to hold the device that is implanted in it, to keep it closed.

For this procedure, your child will be given medication to sleep. Then, in a lab under special x-ray equipment, a team of doctors, nurses, and therapists will pass a tiny catheter into a vein in your child's arm or leg. (Remember, all veins lead to the heart.) While the team watches through the x-ray equipment, the doctor passes the catheter into the right side of the heart. The catheter follows the some path that the blood is taking, and it goes up into the pulmonary artery. By watching on the machines, the doctor can direct the catheter right into the PDA.

Once the catheter is inside the PDA, an umbrellalike device can be inserted into the defect to plug up the shunt. The "umbrella" is coated with material that allows cells to grow on it. When the doctor is satisfied that the placement of the "umbrella" is good, and that it is secure in the PDA, the doctor will release the "umbrella" and remove the catheter. The "umbrella" will act as a barrier to the blood flow. Eventually, the body's natural healing process will allow cells to grow on the "umbrella" and help it seal permanently.

Although it is easier to recover from catheter closure of a PDA than from surgery, it does not come without risks. The "umbrella" that is inserted in the PDA has the potential for breaking free during or immediately after the procedure and entering the blood stream. If this happens, surgery will probably be needed to remove the device and close the PDA. Also, there is the possibility that the "umbrella" will not totally seal the shunt. Again, surgery may also be needed to remove the device and close the PDA to completely stop the blood from shunting.

Some hospitals do catheter closure of PDAs routinely. If your child is recommended for this procedure, find out how long the doctor has been performing it, and what his or her personal statistics are for full recovery without complications. Refer to Chapter 15, "Questions to Ask Your Doctor," for help with this.

SURGERY In the operating room under anesthesia, a PDA can be repaired (Figure 5-2). This is not open heart surgery. The PDA involves the vessels on the outside of the heart, so the heart itself does not need to be cut. Once the child is asleep, the surgeon will make an incision under the left arm, in order to see the pulmonary artery and the aorta. Using two small clamps, one at each end of the PDA, the surgeon will stop the blood from shunting. Then with scissors or a scalpel, the surgeon will cut the vessel between the clamps. Carefully, the cut ends of the shunt are sutured closed, and tied off. By doing this, there is no chance that the PDA will be functional after surgery. The clamps are then removed, and the incision under the arm is closed.

In very small infants, the surgeon may simply tie a few stitches around the PDA, like a tight bow around a package (Figure 5-3). This is usually enough to stop any shunting of blood. It is simply difficult to cut and tie the PDA in a newborn infant because it is too small. Also, the vessels of a newborn infant may not be strong enough to withstand cutting and stitching. Still, if the child has symptoms, it is very important to correct the PDA of even the smallest infants.

What You and Your Child Can Expect in the Future

Today, the risks associated with surgical closure of a PDA are very low. The recovery from surgery is uncomfortable because the incision causes discomfort when moving and coughing. Moving and coughing, however, are both essential for a speedy recovery. Once the PDA is closed, you can expect your child to lead a full normal life.

A Special Note to Parents

In cases where a PDA is not the only congenital heart defect, there might be a good reason to keep the PDA open and shunting blood. With a defect such as Transposition of the Great Vessels, a PDA can be life-saving. Measures can be taken in the very young infant to keep the PDA open until surgery can be performed to correct other defects. This can sometimes be done with an intravenous infusion of prostaglandins, which are hormones known to widen the PDA. However, prostaglandins have a limited power. Often they will not help for more than twenty-four hours after birth, and sometimes less. As always, do not hesitate to communicate directly with your physicians regarding your child's unique situation.

FIGURE 5-2
SURGICAL CORRECTION OF A PDA

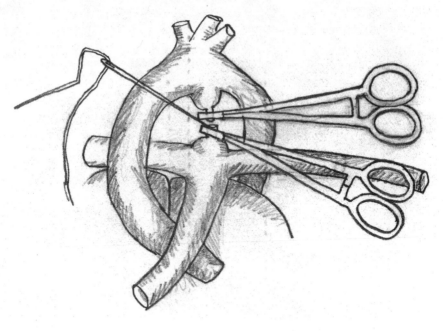

FIGURE 5-3
SURGICAL CORRECTION OF A SMALLER PDA

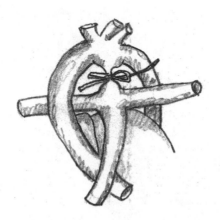

Other Interesting Facts About PDAs

- The first successful surgical closure of a PDA was performed in 1938.
- PDAs occur in approximately 1 of every 2000 full term live births.
- PDAs occur in as high as 75 percent of premature infants born between 28 to 38 weeks of gestation.
- PDAs are more common in females.

CHAPTER 6

Ventricular Septal Defects (VSDs)

A VENTRICULAR SEPTAL DEFECT (VSD) is commonly referred to as a "hole in the heart." As its name explains, it is a defect in the ventricular septum (see Figure 6-1). The ventricles are the larger, bottom chambers in the heart, and they are responsible for forcefully pumping blood out of the heart. The septum is the muscular wall that divides the right and left sides of the heart; the ventricular septal wall separates the right and left ventricles. The ventricular septal wall should be intact; no blood should be able to pass through it. Any opening in the septum that allows blood to cross through it is considered a defect. As a result of the VSD, blood mixes abnormally between the right and the left ventricles.

Since all blood eventually passes through the entire body, you may wonder why mixing blood between the ventricles is considered bad. Remember that the blood in the right and left sides of the heart have different missions. The job of the right ventricle is to pump deoxygenated blood into the pulmonary artery and toward the lungs. When blood reaches the lungs, it gets oxygenated. Blood is then sent from the lungs to the left side of the heart. The job of the left ventricle is to pump that newly oxygenated blood to the body. So, as the right side sends blood to the lungs, the left side sends blood to the body. If any blood gets mixed between the two ventricles, the mixing causes undo stress that requires the heart to work extra hard in order to supply the body with the proper amount of blood flow.

Of the two ventricles, the left ventricle has the hardest job. It has to generate high enough pressure to pump its blood to every part of the body, from your head to your toes. The right ventricle works

FIGURE 6-1
VENTRICULAR SEPTAL DEFECT

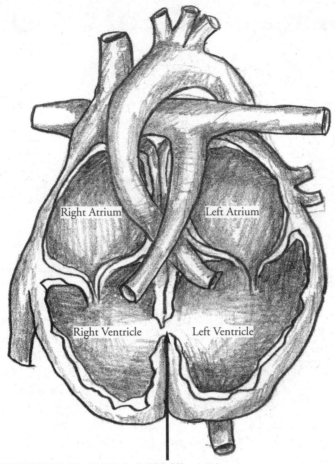

Right Atrium

Left Atrium

Right Ventricle

Left Ventricle

VENTRICULAR SEPTAL DEFECT

at a much lower pressure. Its job is easier because it only has to pump blood to the lungs, which are relatively close to the heart. When the right and left ventricles pump together, the pressures inside their chambers are not equal. The pressure in the left ventricle is much higher than the pressure in the right ventricle.

If there is a hole in the septum, the blood from the left ventricle, under higher pressure, will pump through the defect toward the lower pressure in the right ventricle. This causes two problems:

1. There is now less blood in the left ventricle that is available for the body, so the left ventricle has to work extra hard in order to supply enough blood flow to the arteries of the body.
2. Extra blood in the right ventricle increases its work load. Now it has to pump at a much higher pressure in order to pump the additional blood toward the lungs.

If the VSD is large, there will be a lot of blood crossing over into the right ventricle. Sometimes, the right ventricle and the lungs cannot accommodate this additional flow. As a result, they begin to change. The right ventricle grows bigger and stronger in order to pump the extra blood to the lungs, while the lungs become overwhelmed with the extra flow. The lungs do not want all of that extra blood, so the vessels supplying the lungs tighten up to keep the blood away. The tighter the lungs' blood vessels get, the harder the right ventricle has to work against them. This causes a vicious cycle of higher and higher pressures between the right ventricle and the lungs. If the VSD is not fixed before these pressures get too high, over the years the high pressures in your child's lungs could be the cause of a lot of sickness, including intolerance to activity, constant shortness of breath, and pneumonia.

The size of the defect in the ventricular septum determines how much blood is pumped, or "shunted," through the hole. Naturally, a large VSD will allow a lot of blood to mix from the left side into the right. A small VSD will only allow a little mixing. The more blood that travels across the VSD, the more symptoms your child is likely to experience.

There are many different kinds of VSDs, each classified by its location on the septal wall, and by how many holes there are. Some VSDs are described as being like "Swiss cheese." But most often, VSDs involve only one hole.

The good news is that VSDs do not get bigger; they only get smaller. In fact, 15 to 50 percent of all VSDs will close by themselves within the first few years of a child's life. In general, spontaneous closure of a VSD occurs within the first year of life. After that, there is less of a chance that it will heal on its own, but chances remain, to a smaller degree, until your child reaches three to five years of age. So, if your baby is diagnosed with a small VSD, there may be a 50 percent chance that the defect will close on its own, without medical treatment or surgery.

When a VSD does not close on its own, it is usually due to its size and to its location on the ventricular septum. In fact, VSDs in certain locations on the ventricular septum will never close on their own. So, if your child is having any of the symptoms listed next, your doctor might recommend that the VSD be surgically corrected before age five. Closing the VSD will stop the symptoms from getting worse and will prevent the onset of complications. When your child is tested, ask your doctor specifically if the VSD is in a location where it might close by itself.

Symptoms to Watch For

It is very likely that your child may not have any symptoms at all. In fact, only a small percentage of children with VSDs ever have symptoms. This is mostly because their VSDs are too small to create problems that can be seen outright. Any symptoms that your child may have are directly proportional to the size of the defect and to the amount of blood that mixes from the left to the right ventricle. The larger the defect is, the more mixing will occur, and the more symptoms will appear. But, just because your child may not have symptoms does not mean that you have nothing to worry about. Eventually, the blood that pumps (shunts) through the VSD will cause problems that will negatively affect the heart.

In general, kids who have symptoms usually have larger, or more complicated, defects with a lot of blood mixing between the ventricles. Rapid shallow breathing may be the first sign that something is wrong. Children may have trouble eating because of low energy levels, or because they are constantly trying to catch their breath. Some children will get infections in their lungs. They may also develop a swollen abdomen or an enlarged liver, which can be seen protruding below the rib cage. Most of these symptoms are the result of extra blood flow in the lungs and the high pressures in the right ventricle. If your child begins to develop any symptoms, the child's lung pressures should be monitored closely until surgery can be performed to correct the VSD.

Complications a VSD Can Cause

During the time your child is waiting for surgery, your doctor should be checking frequently to make sure that complications are not developing, and to monitor the size of the VSD to determine whether

Heart Defects in Children

or not the defect is getting smaller. A skilled physician may be able to do this with a stethoscope; the doctor might hear a difference in the intensity of the murmur if it is changing. Or, a test called an *echocardiogram* can be performed to see if the VSD is changing. (Refer to Chapter 13 for an explanation of the echocardiogram.)

Not all children with VSDs will develop complications from the defect. However, those who do generally have been sick and exhibiting symptoms from it. But, children do not have to show symptoms from a VSD before complications arise. Four common complications of a VSD are:

1. infections in the heart;
2. increasingly high blood pressure in the lungs;
3. Pulmonary Vascular Obstructive Disease (caused by the high pressure);
4. damage to the valves in the heart (also caused by the high pressure).

Infections in the Heart

An infection in the heart, and in the valves in the heart, could occur as a complication of a VSD. This is called Bacterial Endocarditis. It is very serious, and your baby can become really sick. (Bacterial Endocarditis is explained fully in Chapter 12.) Children who get Bacterial Endocarditis will be given powerful antibiotics to stop the infection. And, as soon as the infection is cleared up, your doctor may ask that surgery be done to fix the defect and repair any damage that the infection may have caused in the heart. Once the VSD is repaired, the chances that the infection will return are significantly lower.

Increased Pressure in the Lungs

If the VSD is large and a lot of blood crosses over into the right ventricle, abnormally high pressures can develop in your baby's heart and lungs. Your doctor can tell if high pressures in the lungs are developing through tests such as a cardiac catheterization (which is described in Chapter 13). If high lung pressures develop, they cause a vicious cycle of higher and higher pressures between the right ventricle and the lungs. Fortunately, they do not usually get to the point of being irreversible for a few years.

Pulmonary Vascular Obstructive Disease

If the VSD is not fixed before pressures in the lungs get too high, a condition called Pulmonary Vascular Obstructive Disease can occur. This condition develops because of years of pressure buildup between the right ventricle and the lungs. A cycle of higher and higher pressures makes it almost impossible for the heart to pump blood into the lungs—blood gets trapped in the right ventricle and cannot get into the lungs. Since no oxygen exchange can occur, a child could die. Fortunately, it takes a long time to develop Pulmonary Vascular Obstructive Disease (the final stages of this disease usually do not happen until the child reaches adulthood). However, because of this serious complication of a VSD, every child should be closely monitored for rising lung pressures. If high lung pressures begin to develop, surgery will be necessary.

Damage to the Heart's Valves

The fourth complication resulting from a VSD is damage to any of the four valves in the heart. Damage to the valves happens because of the high pressures that develop in the heart, and the turbulent flow of blood through the VSD, which can cause stress on valves. When this happens, the valves stretch and widen. This causes incomplete closure of the valve, and blood leaks through it even when it is closed. If valve damage occurs, your child's doctor may have to surgically correct both the VSD and the valve.

Medical Treatment You Can Expect
Medications

There is no medicine that will fix a VSD. If the defect is going to close on its own it will (15 to 50 percent do), whether your child is on medication or not. However, your doctor will prescribe medicine to treat any symptoms that develop, and to delay surgery until your child reaches an acceptable age for surgical repair. If your infant is very sick but can be treated with medicine until six months of age, surgery can be held off until then. But, if medicine fails to keep the infant healthy and growing, surgery may need to be done before six months.

Three common medications that your child may need are:
- antibiotics to treat or prevent respiratory infections;
- Digoxin to help the heart contract strongly and evenly; and
- Lasix to prevent extra fluid buildup in the body.

The appendix on pages 137 through 139 provides a brief explanation of some common medications and what they are used for.

Surgery

WHEN IT'S NEEDED If your child is exhibiting symptoms even while on medication, or if complications are beginning to arise, surgery may be indicated. Surgery should also be done if there is no change in the size of your child's vsd by the age of three or four, even if the child doesn't have any symptoms. This is because with every passing year there is more risk for complications to develop, and they are too serious to ignore.

If your baby is very young and has symptoms, surgery may be needed within the first three months. If the child can stay healthy with medicine and proper nutrition, however, surgery can sometimes be postponed until approximately six months, a time when the risks of surgery are much lower. Children who are very sick at a young age because of large vsds have very little chance of the defect closing on its own.

THE PROCEDURE All children, even young babies, are given total anesthesia so that they are asleep through the entire operation. Once the child is under anesthesia, the surgeon will make an incision in the center of the chest in order to see the heart. The actual procedure for fixing a vsd is similar to mending. Some small holes are simply stitched closed, just as you would sew together a small tear in your clothes. A larger defect may require a patch to cover the hole. There are different kinds of patches that can be used. The most common is a piece of the child's own tissue, which is taken from the pericardium and sutured over the hole in the septum. The pericardium is a protective, skinlike sac that covers the heart. Because it is part of the growing body, this piece of tissue is perfect for fixing the hole. Growing muscle fibers on the septum will mesh with the patch, and it will grow with the child's heart.

There are man-made patches that can also be used to repair a vsd. These patches are all made of a sterile, sturdy fabric, and they are sutured over the hole much like a knee patch is added to a pair of trousers. Growing muscle fibers in the heart will mesh with these sterile patches as part of the body's natural healing process. The heart's tissue will grow to help seal the septum and provide a smooth surface where there once was a hole.

How long the surgery will take depends on what kind of patch is used and how involved the repair is. Your child's recovery will be uncomfortable because the incision will hurt when the child moves or coughs. Moving and coughing, however, are both a very important part of a speedy recovery. After this open heart surgery, your child will be put on antibiotics to prevent infections, and possibly other medicines immediately after surgery. Usually, these medications are used to help the body recover from surgery and to help the heartbeat stay strong. (A complete guide to the day of surgery is provided in Chapter 14.)

What You and Your Child Can Expect in the Future

Once the VSD is fixed, if there are no complications, you can expect your child to lead a full normal, healthy life without limitations. There are, however, risks associated with open heart surgery. Your doctor will review these risks in specifics with you before the surgery occurs. Since the risks of surgical closure of a VSD are estimated to be very low—approximately 1 to 2 percent—you and your child can feel reassured about having the surgery.

A Special Note to Parents

Sometimes after surgery your doctor will impose physical restrictions on your child to ensure a smooth recovery. Every situation is different. Be direct and specific when you speak with your doctor. Ask if the child's activities will be limited for a month, a year, or forever. Find out if the doctors mean to limit running and playing; usually they do not. Be sure to get a time frame—the doctor may mean no running and playing for just this month. As always, do not hesitate to communicate directly with your physicians regarding your child's unique situation.

Interesting Facts About VSDs

- VSDs are the most commonly recognized congenital heart defects.
- VSDs occur in about two of every one thousand live babies born today.
- VSDs occur with approximately 50 percent of all other kinds of congenital heart defects.

Heart Defects in Children

CHAPTER 7

Aortic Stenosis

THE AORTA IS THE largest artery in the body. It carries newly oxygenated blood from the left ventricle in the heart to the body. This blood is then able to fuel the muscles with oxygen and nutrients, which are needed for growth and energy. A stenosis in the aorta is a narrowing of the vessel, which limits the amount of blood flow that can get through to the body (Figure 7-1). There are different types of stenosis that can occur in the aorta. The two main types are Stenosis of the Aortic Valve and Stenosis of the Aorta.

Stenosis of the Aortic Valve

The most common kind of Aortic Stenosis your child can have is a Stenosis of the Aortic Valve. Normally, the aortic valve easily opens and closes to control the flow of blood from the left ventricle to the body. When the valve is stenotic, it is rigid against the flow of blood through it. This rigidity forces the left ventricle to work extra hard in order to pump blood through the stenotic valve. The left ventricle must generate higher pressures to move an adequate amount of blood flow through the valve and to the body. The more stenosis there is in the aortic valve, the higher resistance there will be to the blood flow through it, and the harder the heart will have to work to get oxygenated blood to the tissues and organs of the body.

Stenosis of the Aorta

If there is no problem with your child's aortic valve, there may be a narrowing of the passage of blood before or after the area of the valve. (Also see Chapter 8, "Coarctation of the Aorta.") In this case, as with stenosis of the valve itself, the left ventricle must generate

FIGURE 7-1
AORTIC STENOSIS AT THE VALVE

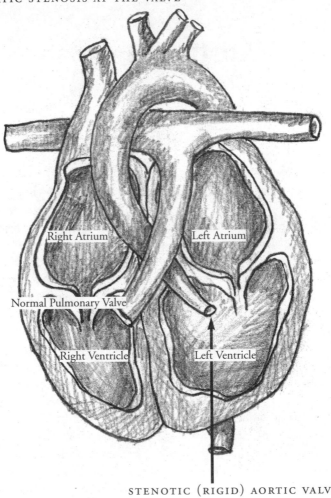

Right Atrium

Left Atrium

Normal Pulmonary Valve

Right Ventricle

Left Ventricle

STENOTIC (RIGID) AORTIC VALVE

higher pressures in order to move an adequate amount of blood through the narrowing in the aorta to the body. The narrower the passageway is, the higher the resistance will be to the blood flow across the stricture, and the harder the heart will have to work to get oxygenated blood to the tissues and organs of the body.

Over a period of time, if the left ventricle is forced to work extra hard, problems can arise. The harder the heart works, the more oxygen it needs. And, just like any other muscle in your body, when you work it hard, it bulks up. (Doctors call this condition *hypertrophy*.) Body builders like it, but increasing the muscle thickness in the heart is not desirable. The thicker the muscle is, the harder it works, and the more oxygen it requires to function properly. The larger the heart becomes, the more oxygen it needs. Often, the body cannot keep up with the increasing oxygen demands of the heart. This is bad because if the heart does not get enough oxygen, it can cause pain in the heart (called *angina*). Pain from the heart muscle because of a low oxygen supply to the heart is dangerous, and it can lead to abnormal heart rhythms.

Even if your child's aortic valve is functioning well and without problems, a stenosis in the aorta may put extra stress on the valve and cause damage to it. The high pressures that are generated by the left ventricle to eject blood past the stenotic area in the aorta may damage the integrity of the aortic valve itself, and produce leaks. A leak will prevent even more blood from being able to get through to the body. If this happens, the left ventricle will have to generate even higher pressures to send enough of the oxygenated blood supply to the body where it is needed for growth and energy.

A child with Aortic Stenosis has an interruption in the flow of blood to the body. Since the aorta is carrying oxygenated blood to the body, the body can become deprived of oxygen, and this is of great concern. How can the body function normally if there is not enough oxygen in its tissues? Sometimes it cannot.

Symptoms to Watch For

In severe cases of Aortic Stenosis, some infants and young children may have problems with irritability and poor weight gain. The irritability can be caused by heart pain (angina), or by fatigue from the energy that the heart is expending to oxygenate the body. Heart pain will usually occur during feeding, and uncontrollable crying might be the first sign that your child is having pain. The stenosis in the aorta makes the heart work extra hard in order to pump an adequate amount of blood supply to your child's body. Because of this, all of the energy that the child may have used to play, laugh, and grow is used up by the heart. This may make the child very tired. Poor weight gain in these children is due to the lack of energy the body has. If a lot of energy is being used by the heart, there is very little left for digestion and growth.

Your child may have a fast heartbeat, pale or cool skin, and cyanosis (blueness of the skin, lips, or nails). Stenosis in the aorta decreases the amount of blood that goes to the body with each contraction of the heart, so the heart begins to pump faster in order to increase the amount of flow. This process is called a "compensatory mechanism." Basically, it means that the heart is compensating for the low amount of blood flow around the body. The faster the heart beats, the more blood it can expel. Unfortunately, this mechanism is not foolproof. When the heart beats faster than it should, it does not give itself enough time to "fill up" between beats. So, it may not be pumping at its full capacity. The body recognizes this and makes the heart beat even faster to compensate for the low volume in the heart. This process becomes a vicious cycle, and eventually the heart muscle will fatigue and may become painful.

The decreased amount of blood flow in the body may cause the skin to become pale, cool, or cyanotic (blue). Remember, blood carries oxygen and nutrients to the tissues and organs in the body. If the blood supply is low, the oxygen levels are also low. Low oxygen levels in the body cause the bluish appearance of the skin. But before this happens, your child's skin may first become pale or cool. Luckily, our bodies are very smart. Our brains can sense low blood flow and low oxygen levels in our bodies. When it does, it makes the arteries and veins constrict or squeeze, to divert any extra blood away from the fingers and toes to the brain and major organs of the body. This way, the brain and organs do not suffer from low blood flow or low oxygen levels. That is why the skin gets pale and cool. The blood that should make it pink and warm is being sent to more important places. This is a good "compensatory mechanism," because it manages to keep the brain and other organs of the body healthy.

An older child who slowly develops Aortic Stenosis seems to do better than an infant who has it and has already been diagnosed. This is mostly because of the severity of the defect. If it is detected early in infancy, it is generally more severe than if it is not noticed until the child has grown. All of the same symptoms and complications may develop as a result of the defect, but the symptoms come on much more gradually. When the symptoms occur slowly, doctors have more time to diagnose the problem and plan the best care possible for your child.

Heart Defects in Children

Complications Aortic Stenosis Can Cause

If any of the following complications develop, it is very important to correct your child's stenosis. Ideally, Aortic Stenosis should be corrected before any of these complications arise. But, appropriate steps must be taken by the medical staff to ensure that your child will get to the operating room in the healthiest condition possible. If complications arise, or if your child is becoming undernourished because of poor feeding, the doctor may hospitalize the child for treatment before the operation itself.

Angina

Severe cases of Aortic Stenosis can lead to angina (heart pain). This is bad because when the heart hurts it is usually the result of ischemia. Ischemia means that there is not enough oxygen available to meet the needs of the busy heart. Pain from ischemia is the body's way of saying "slow down." But, since the heart cannot slow down, ischemia can lead to abnormal heart rhythms.

Congestive Heart Failure

Children and infants who have very severe cases of Aortic Stenosis can develop symptoms of congestive heart failure. This is a condition caused by a "backup" of blood in the body because of increased pressures in the heart. The child may be short of breath or may breathe shallowly and rapidly. The child may have swelling in the legs or abdomen and may develop frequent respiratory infections.

Heart Valve Problems

If your child's Aortic Stenosis goes uncorrected, it can lead to problems in adulthood. Uncorrected Aortic Stenosis, even if your child is not sick or does not have symptoms, may lead to heart valve problems. This is because of years of high-pressured blood flow in the heart and through the valve. Blood that ejects through the valves at high pressures can cause damage and incomplete closure of the valves. If damage occurs, the valve may eventually need surgical correction.

Heart Attacks

Adults who have uncorrected Aortic Stenosis have an increased risk of heart attacks. The enlarged heart muscle cannot continually function without an adequate supply of oxygen. When it is forced to, it needs more and more oxygen to survive. If these demands for oxygen are not met, parts of the muscle can starve and/or die. This is what happens during a heart attack, which can be painful and deadly.

Treatment You Can Expect
Medications
There is no medicine that will cure a stenosis of the aorta or the aortic valve. Any medicine that is used will be to prevent, or control, any symptoms or complications that may develop. An infant with severe Aortic Stenosis may be fed through a small feeding tube prior to surgery, to promote weight gain. The feeding tube is used to decrease energy expenditure; if the child does not have to suck to get food, energy is saved that can be used for growth. Healthy tissues and fat stores are used by the body to heal wounds. So, adequate weight gain and proper nutrition are particularly important before surgery.

Medicine is used to control symptoms of congestive heart failure and abnormal heart rhythms. Some common medications that your child may be on might include:

- Lasix to prevent swelling in the body and to control mucous in the lungs;
- Digoxin to help the heart contract strongly and evenly;
- Vitamins to help with growth and nutrition.

Your child may be on other medications as well. Refer to pages 137 through 139 for a more detailed explanation of some commonly used medications.

Surgery
All children, even young babies, are given total anesthesia so that they are asleep through the entire operation. Once the child is under anesthesia, the surgeon will make an incision in the front of the chest in order to see the heart and its vessels. The aortic valve can be either repaired or replaced.

REPAIRING THE AORTIC VALVE The repair of a stenotic aortic valve may only involve the snipping of the leaflets. Leaflets open and close to allow blood to flow through the valve (Figure 7-2). Some-

FIGURE 7-2

THE AORTIC VALVE

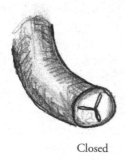
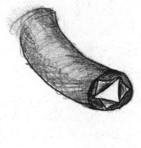

Closed   Open

times, stenosis is caused by the leaflets' inability to open. If they get "stuck together," blood cannot get through. The surgeon can make a cut between the leaflets where they are naturally supposed to open. Once this is done, the valve should work normally. This procedure is called an "Aortic Valve Commissurotomy."

If the aortic valve functions normally, but the opening for the valve is small (Figure 7-1), the surgeon can make an incision on the outside of the aorta to widen the area around the valve. Once the area is widened, a small patch can be sewn over that area of the valve to make it larger. This releases the narrowing of the valve area. Once the area is opened wider, blood can flow more freely through the valve into the aorta. This procedure can also be used if there is a stenosis on the aorta directly after the area of the valve.

REPLACING THE AORTIC VALVE If the aortic valve itself is damaged, or if there is a more complicated repair needed to ensure proper flow of blood across the valve, the surgeon may choose to replace the valve. Aortic valve replacement in a young child is only done if the other procedures mentioned here will not work. This is mostly because if children need a new valve at a very young age, as they grow, the replaced valve may become too small, and it will need to be replaced again at other intervals in the children's life. Sometimes the replacement of your child's aortic valve may eventually be necessary some years after a repair is done.

There are many kinds of mechanical and tissue valves that are used today to replace a child's damaged valve. A mechanical valve is made in a laboratory by scientists. It is built to function most closely like a human valve should. A tissue valve is usually taken from an animal, and most commonly from the aorta of a pig. Pigs have very similar hearts to people, and their heart valves have been used a lot. Your surgeon will use whichever valve he or she is most comfortable with, making sure to choose the valve that will produce the best results for your child's recovery. The use of an artificial valve may require your child to be on lifelong medication to thin the blood. Tissue valves, as a rule, do not require blood-thinning medications, but they tend to have a shorter life span, and they may need to be replaced sooner than the mechanical valves. Remember that every child's defect is different. The valve that one child may have received might not be the right one for your child. Your doctor will know how to help you choose the proper treatment for your child.

Replacing the aortic valve requires the surgeon to cut the existing valve out. Once it is removed, the replacement valve is carefully sutured into place. The incision that was made on the aorta (to get to the valve) is closed with stitches and the replacement is complete.

FIXING STENOSIS ON THE AORTA In the operating room under anesthesia, a stenosis of the aorta can be repaired. Once your child is asleep, the surgeon will make an incision in the center of the chest in order to see the heart and its vessels. Stenosis on the aorta is sometimes referred to as an "Hourglass Deformity" because the defect in the vessel looks very similar to an hourglass (Figure 7-3). If the stenosis occurs high above the valve, these defects are called "Coarctation of the Aorta." (Refer to Chapter 8 for a more detailed explanation of Coarctation of the Aorta.)

Repair of an "Hourglass Deformity" on the aorta requires a vertical incision through the defect itself (Figure 7-4). Once the narrowed area is opened from the incision through the area, a patch is carefully sewn on it. This patch serves to widen the deformity and to keep the vessel open for blood to flow more easily through it and to the body.

If there is a restriction to blood flow below the valve, it usually involves muscle thickening in the heart itself, or the growth of additional membranes around the opening of the valve (Figure 7-3). These things cause obstruction of flow through the normally

FIGURE 7-3
AORTIC STENOSIS ABOVE AND BELOW THE VALVE

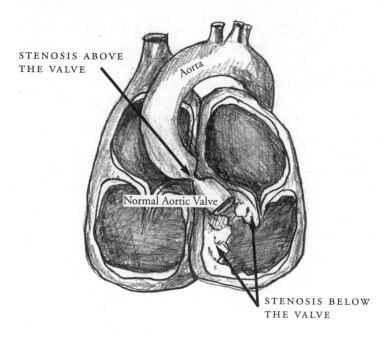

STENOSIS ABOVE
THE VALVE

Aorta

Normal Aortic Valve

STENOSIS BELOW
THE VALVE

FIGURE 7-4
STENOSIS ON THE AORTA

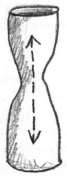

Vertical Incision

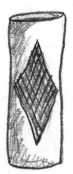

Patch to widen
the aorta

Aortic Stenosis

functioning valves and the aorta. In this case, the surgeon may just need to cut the obstructive area out and take it away from the valve.

What You and Your Child Can Expect in the Future

Please keep in mind that every child is different. No two children with the same defect will react to treatment the same way. This is mostly because every person's anatomy is slightly different than the next. The results of operations for children with Aortic Stenosis are good.

Approximately 50 to 60 percent of children who have a repair of their valve done, without replacement, need to go back for another operation to repair again, or replace, their valve within about twenty years. This is mostly because the valve gets stenotic again. Even though the valve may need additional surgery, it is still very important for you to consider the initial surgical correction of these defects. The long-term complications of uncorrected Aortic Stenosis in most cases outweigh the surgical risks.

If your child receives a mechanical valve as replacement of the aortic valve, you can expect the child to be on lifelong medication to thin the blood. This is done to make sure that the artificial valve does not destroy the blood cells as it opens and closes. Thinning the blood makes the cells "slippery" and lowers their chances of getting squashed in the valve when it closes. Blood thinning also reduces the risk of forming blood clots that can cause strokes or heart attacks. However, your child will bruise and bleed easily. Because of this, the child may not be allowed to play contact sports, which may cause hidden injuries, such as internal bleeding. If your child is put on blood thinners, frequent blood tests called "bleeding times" (or "PTS") will be done to regulate the dosage of the medication.

A Special Note to Parents

Speak with your physician about the need for antibiotics throughout the child's life. An infection called Endocarditis can occur in the heart valves when there is a defect, or when surgery has been performed in the heart. (Refer to Chapter 12 on Bacterial Endocarditis.) Some doctors will prescribe antibiotics to be taken before any surgical procedure, especially including dental work. Endocarditis can damage the valves, and another operation might be needed to repair them.

Heart Defects in Children

According to the current literature on heart defects, approximately one in five children with Aortic Stenosis will have at least one other defect. Be certain that your child has been thoroughly tested. If another defect is present, ask your doctor if the surgeons can fix it when they correct the stenosis. Otherwise, a second operation may be needed.

Interesting Facts About Aortic Stenosis

- Aortic Stenosis occurs in approximately 3 to 10 percent of all children with congenital heart defects.
- Approximately 60 to 75 percent of children with Aortic Stenosis have an obstruction at the valve.
- Approximately one in five children with Aortic Stenosis has at least one other cardiac defect present.
- The most common associated defects with Aortic Stenosis include:
    a.) Patent Ductus Arteriosus (Chapter 5);
    b.) Coarctation of the Aorta (Chapter 8);
    c.) Ventricular Septal Defect (Chapter 6);
    d.) Stenosis of the Mitral Valve (Chapter 11); and
    e.) Hypoplastic Left Heart Syndrome (Chapter 11).

Coarctation of the Aorta

THE AORTA IS THE largest artery in the body. It carries freshly oxygenated blood from the left ventricle, in the heart, to the body. This blood is then used to fuel our muscles with oxygen and nutrients that are needed for growth and energy. Coarctation of the Aorta is a lot like Aortic Stenosis (see Chapter 7). A coarctation is a narrowing in the aorta that slows down the normal flow of blood out of the heart into the body. Unlike Aortic Stenosis, the narrowing caused by Coarctation of the Aorta occurs on the aortic arch. The aortic arch is the area where the aorta "arches" up and curves over the top of the heart. Then, the aorta descends into the body (Figure 8-1).

Coarctation of the Aorta is a stricture in the vessel that acts like a tight rubber band around a straw. It is a deformity that looks like an hourglass. How severe the defect is depends mostly on how narrow the stricture on the vessel becomes. As a child grows, the aorta grows too, but the rubber band-like defect around the aorta stays tight. The more a child grows, the more freshly oxygenated blood the body needs from the aorta. (Remember, oxygen and nutrients found in the blood are essential to fuel the muscles and tissues for growth.) But, even as the child grows, the band around the aorta stays tight. This means that less blood can get through to the body.

The heart will begin to pump stronger and faster if there is not enough blood getting through to the body. As this happens, blood is even more forcefully ejected up into the aorta. However, the blood does not make it down into the body. There are three arteries that rise out of the aorta at the top of the aortic arch (Figure 8-1). These three arteries carry blood to the brain and the upper body. Because there is a narrowing in the aorta just below these arteries, blood

FIGURE 8-1
COARCTATION OF THE AORTA

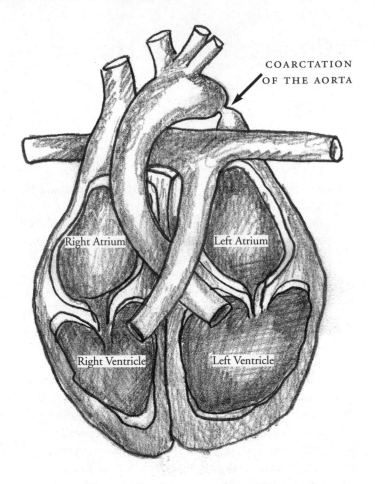

COARCTATION
OF THE AORTA

Right Atrium

Left Atrium

Right Ventricle

Left Ventricle

flow from the heart is forced up into them. As the heart pumps, they get flooded with blood.

With an increase in blood flow to the upper body through the three arteries, high blood pressure will develop in that area. At the same time, the lower body is not getting the same amount of blood flow. It has low blood pressure. Consequently, the heart has to work harder and harder to get adequate blood flow to the legs and abdomen. Blood pressure in the arms and head gets very high, but it stays low in the legs and abdomen.

Symptoms to Watch For

Infants and very young children with Coarctation of the Aorta will have problems with irritability and poor weight gain. According to recent medical literature, approximately one half of all infants born with this defect will experience symptoms within the first few months of life. Irritability can be caused by heart pain (angina) or fatigue. Heart pain usually happens during feeding, and uncontrollable crying can be the first sign.

The narrowing in the aorta causes the heart to work extra hard in order to pump an adequate amount of blood to your child's body. Because of this, all of the energy the body may have used to laugh, play, and grow is used up by the heart. Because of this, your child may be very tired. Poor weight gain in children with Coarctation of the Aorta is due to the lack of energy the body has for growth. Poor eating is due to pain, rapid breathing, and fatigue. If a lot of energy is being used by the heart, there is very little left for digestion and growth.

Your child may have a fast heartbeat, rapid breathing, and pale, cool skin in the lower body. If the Coarctation of the Aorta is severe, it may even cause cyanosis (blueness) of the lower body. This is because of the decrease in the amount of blood going to the legs and abdomen. But at the same time, the arms, face, and upper body may be warm and even flushed or pink.

The heart beats fast in order to make up for the low amount of blood flow to the lower body. The faster the heart beats, the more blood it can expel. Unfortunately, when this happens, it may not give itself enough time to fill up between contractions. Consequently, it may be pumping at less than its full capacity. The body recognizes this, and makes the heart beat even faster to make up for the low blood flow. This process becomes a vicious cycle. Eventually, the heart muscle fatigues, and it can become painful.

The more blood the heart beats into the aorta, the more blood flow there is to the head and upper extremities. This will cause abnormal "overdevelopment" of the head, chest, and arms. This kind of development looks exaggerated when compared to the "underdevelopment" of the hips and legs. In addition, your child may have strong pulses in the arms and neck, while the hips and legs will have very weak pulses. This is sometimes the first telltale sign that there is a Coarctation of the Aorta.

Complications a Coarctation of the Aorta Can Cause
Small Growth of the Lower Extremities
Low blood pressure in the legs and abdomen can cause small growth of the lower extremities. A child with Coarctation of the aorta may develop small, thin legs, and a large upper body.

Angina
Severe cases of Coarctation of the Aorta can lead to angina (heart pain). This is bad because when the heart hurts, it is the result of ischemia. Ischemia means that there is not enough oxygen available to meet the needs of the busy heart. Pain from ischemia is the body's way of saying "slow down." But, since the heart cannot slow down, ischemia can cause abnormal heart rhythms.

Inadequate Blood Flow to the Lower Body
To compensate for the narrowing in the aorta, the heart has to pump extra hard to get an adequate amount of blood to flow to the lower body. The stricture in the vessel acts like a barrier to blood flow. The heart, just like any other muscle in your body, will bulk up if you work it out. (Doctors call this condition hypertrophy.) But the increase in muscle thickness in the heart is not desirable. The thicker the muscle is, the more oxygen it requires to function properly. If the heart does not get enough oxygen, angina (heart pain) and abnormal heart rhythms can occur.

A child with Coarctation of the Aorta has an interruption in the flow of blood to the lower body. Since the aorta carries oxygenated blood to the body, the lower body can become deprived of oxygen. This is of great concern. How can the body function normally if there is not enough oxygen? Sometimes it cannot.

Congestive Heart Failure
Children with Coarctation of the Aorta can also develop symptoms of congestive heart failure. This condition is characterized by a swollen abdomen and frequent respiratory infections. Basically, it is a "backup" of blood in the body because of the increased pressure in the heart that is caused by the narrowing in the aorta. This can cause swelling that can be seen particularly in the legs and abdomen, and in some children it may cause shortness of breath.

Heart Defects in Children

High Blood Pressure and Kidney Failure

If Coarctation of the Aorta goes uncorrected, and there is low blood flow to the lower body, problems with the kidneys can develop. The kidneys help to filter out waste products from the blood. Urine is made in the kidneys and excreted through the bladder. When there is not enough blood getting to the kidneys, they react violently. The kidneys can eventually excrete enzymes that cause very high blood pressure in the body. The higher the kidneys can make the blood pressure, the more likely they are to get the blood flow they need. High blood pressure of this nature can be dangerous because it can cause strokes and heart attacks. But, if the kidneys do not get enough blood flow, they can go into kidney failure. This means that the kidneys can no longer work, and they may eventually need the help of dialysis machines to clean the blood.

Aneurysm of the Aorta

Uncorrected Coarctation of the Aorta can also have other devastating complications. An aneurysm on the aorta can develop because of years of very high pressure in the aorta. An aneurysm is a weakening in the wall of the aorta from constant pounding from the blood's pressure on the vessel. The weak portion of the vessel can out-patch. If the weakened vessel ruptures, it can cause death.

Strokes

Strokes can also occur in adults with this uncorrected defect. Strokes happen as the result of years of very high blood pressure in the head. Remember, the coarctation usually sits below the three arteries that bring blood to the upper body. So, as blood enters the aorta, it gets forcefully expelled into these arteries. Years of high velocity blood flow can cause weakening in the arteries of the head. If these arteries rupture, bleeding from them can cause strokes.

Medical Treatment You Can Expect
Medications

Medical treatment of Coarctation of the Aorta is aimed directly at preventing and controlling symptoms and complications. Before surgery, an infant with a severe coarctation might be fed through a feeding tube to promote weight gain. The feeding tube is used to decrease energy expenditure; if the child does not have to suck to get food, energy is saved. That energy can be used for growth. Healthy tissues and fat stores are used by the body to heal wounds. So, adequate weight gain is particularly important before surgery.

Medicine is used to control symptoms of congestive heart failure and high blood pressure (hypertension). Some common medications that your child may be on might include:

- Lasix to prevent swelling in the body and to control mucous in the lungs;
- Digoxin to help the heart contract strongly and evenly;
- Vitamins to help with growth and nutrition.

Your child may also be on other medications. Refer to pages 137 through 139 for an explanation of some commonly used medications.

Mechanical Ventilation

Very sick infants and children might need help breathing. Sometimes, mechanical ventilation with tubes and machines is necessary to keep the child safely breathing before surgery can be performed to correct the defect.

Surgery

All children, even young babies, are given total anesthesia so that they are asleep through the entire operation. Once the child is under anesthesia, Coarctation of the Aorta can be corrected. After your child is asleep, the surgeon will make an incision down the front of the chest in order to see the heart and its vessels. Some surgeons will use a thoracotomy incision, which goes under the left arm and across to the back. You will want to ask your doctors which approach they will use. A thoracotomy incision can be more cosmetically pleasing, especially in girls.

There are several approaches to correcting the defect on the aorta. One way to fix the narrowing on the aorta is by cutting out the affected area and sewing the aorta back together (Figure 8-2). Clamps are placed on the aorta at both ends of the defect. The aorta is cut between the clamps, the defect is removed, and the two ends are sewn together. This procedure is called an "end-to-end anastomosis." It is a good procedure because it removes all of the abnormal tissue in the defect. But, it may be a technically difficult operation to perform because of the location of the defect. The coarctation can be very close to the arteries that come from the aorta. The surgeon has

FIGURE 8-2
END-TO-END ANASTOMOSIS

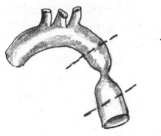
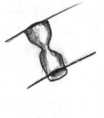
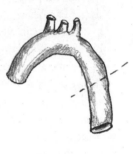

2. Affected area is excised.	2. Affected area is discarded.	3. Remaining portions are connected.

to be very careful not to damage those vessels. This surgery generally takes longer than other approaches. Many children will have postoperative complications associated with long operations. For this
reason, some doctors will choose a different surgical technique.

Similar to the end-to-end anastomosis procedure is a technique
involving a tubelike implant on the aorta. When the defective area
is cut off the vessel, the surgeon can implant a sterile tube onto the
aorta to replace it (Figure 8-3). This approach has its limitations, however. The patch cannot grow with the child. This is of concern because subsequent operations are sometimes necessary to enlarge the
tube as the aorta grows.

FIGURE 8-3
COARCTATION CORRECTED WITH AN IMPLANT

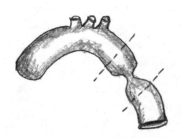
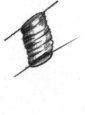
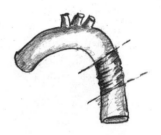

Surgeons may elect to use a patch to correct Coarctation of the Aorta. This procedure is identical to the patch repair of Aortic Stenosis (refer to Chapter 7, Figure 7-4). Patches are made of a sterile, sturdy material that can withstand the high-pressured blood flow in the aorta. In this case, a clamp is used to temporarily stop the flow of blood in the aorta. An incision is made down through the narrowing in the vessel, and an oval patch is then sewn into the incision. By adding the surface area of the patch to the aorta, the defect is widened. Some surgeons like this approach better than the end-to-end anastomosis because it works well, and it is quicker to perform. When operations can be performed without long operating times, there are typically fewer complications. And, because the patch does not encompass the entire diameter of the aorta, the vessel can usually grow and expand with age.

Some institutions are currently doing research with "Balloon Angioplasty" of Coarctation of the Aorta. This procedure is not an operation, so it can be performed in a Cardiac Cath Lab. It involves a catheter with a deflated balloon that is inserted into the aorta under special x-ray equipment. Doctors can see the area of the aorta that is narrowed. The balloon is opened up and squashed against the narrowed area in the aorta to enlarge it. This procedure is very new in the treatment of coarctation. Early results of these studies reveal many complications, including tearing of the aorta, bleeding in the aorta, aneurysm formation at the site of repair, scaring of the vessel, and restenosis of the aorta (the vessel narrows again after the procedure). However, these studies are still in the early stages of development. If perfected, they may eventually prove to be a reasonable alternative to surgery.

After surgical repair of this defect, children may need additional medication to keep their blood pressure normal. High blood pressure in the immediate postoperative period is dangerous to the repair. Stitches that are used on the aorta can tear if the blood pressure gets too high. Your child may also be put on other medications immediately after surgery. Usually, they are used to help the body recover. Refer to pages 137 through 139 for more detailed explanations of medications you may encounter.

What You and Your Child Can Expect in the Future

Please keep in mind that every child is different. No two children with the same defect will react to treatment the same way. This is mostly because every person's anatomy is slightly different than the next. Still, the results of operations for children with a Coarctation of the Aorta are good.

Studies of patients with corrected Coarctation of the Aorta over the long term show that most of the complications in adulthood were from high blood pressure. It was found that if the children did not have high blood pressure for a long period of time before the initial repair, they did much better through adulthood. So, early repair of this defect is strongly recommended. The best long-term health results were obtained from children whose defects were repaired between the ages of one and four.

A Special Note to Parents

Frequently, the need for a second, and sometimes third, operation will arise. This is mostly because of restenosis of the vessel. The tissue on the aorta surrounding the coarctation can sometimes continue to grow defectively. If this happens, there may be a need to reoperate to stop any narrowing that may occur as a result. Another major cause for a reoperation would be to enlarge a tube graft or patch that may have been inserted if your child was very young at the time of the repair. As children grow, the aorta grows, but patches and grafts do not.

There is a strong possibility that other defects can be present with Coarctation of the Aorta. Be certain that your child has been thoroughly tested. If another defect is present, the surgeons should fix it when they correct the coarctation. This may eliminate the need for additional surgery.

Interesting Facts About Coarctation of the Aorta
- Coarctation of the Aorta is the eighth most common congenital heart defect.
- An estimated one in every twelve hundred live births will have a Coarctation of the Aorta.
- Boys are more commonly affected than girls (two to five times more often).

- Coarctation was first diagnosed in a child in 1835, but there was no correction for the defect way back then.
- Coarctation of the Aorta can be suspected in any patients who have high blood pressure under the age of fifty, especially if they have muscular upper bodies but small hips and legs.
- The first successful surgical repair of Coarctation of the Aorta was reported in 1945 by two doctors named Craaford and Nylin.

CHAPTER 9

Tetralogy of Fallot

IN 1888, a French physician named Dr. E. Fallot first discovered and published his findings about this condition. As its name suggests, it actually involves four defects in the heart. These defects can occur separately, but when all four defects occur together, they form the classic characteristics of Tetralogy of Fallot. Tetralogy of Fallot is commonly referred to as "Tetralogy," or simply "Tet." Tetralogy can be difficult to understand. Review this chapter slowly, and refer frequently to the pictures.

There are four defects that characterize Tetralogy:
1. Ventricular Septal Defect (VSD) (see Chapter 6);
2. Aortic Overriding (the opening of the aorta is directly over the defect in the ventricular septum);
3. Right Ventricular Outflow Tract Obstruction (obstruction to blood flow out of the right ventricle);
4. Right Ventricular Hypertrophy (abnormal enlargement of the muscular walls of the right ventricle).

It is almost hard to believe that these four defects can occur together so consistently. Surprisingly, all four defects are the result of one developmental inconsistency; the septum (wall) that divides the right and left ventricles is misaligned.

Ventricular Septal Defect
As we discussed in Chapter 2, the ventricles are the large chambers at the bottom of the heart. They are responsible for pumping blood to the lungs (from the right ventricle) and to the body (from the left ventricle). The right and left ventricles are separated by the ventricular septum. This wall should be intact, and no blood should be

able to pass through it. A defect, or hole, in the septum will allow abnormal mixing of blood between the two sides of the heart.

Because all blood eventually goes through the entire body, you may wonder why mixing right- and left-sided blood is considered bad. Remember that the blood in the right ventricle is low in oxygen. It gets pumped into the pulmonary artery toward the lungs to be oxygenated. But blood in the left ventricle has just come from the lungs. That blood is rich with oxygen, and it is ready to be pumped to the body to be used as energy. So, the right and left sides of the heart have different missions. Any mixing of blood between the ventricles can cause unnecessary stress on the body. For a better understanding of Ventricular Septal Defects, please refer to Chapter 6.

Aortic Overriding

With this condition, the wall between the ventricles not only is misaligned, it also leans a little toward the right. This tiny rotation of the septal wall places the defect in the Ventricular Septum (VSD) directly under the aorta (see Figure 9-1). The aorta is the largest artery in the body. It carries freshly oxygenated blood from the left ventricle in the heart to the body. The body uses this freshly oxygenated blood for food and fuel. If there is a hole in the wall between the right and left ventricles, and the aorta is moved over the hole, there is trouble. When the ventricles pump, blood from both sides of the heart is ejected up into the aorta. This means that the body is getting some of the blood that should be going to the lungs for oxygen. This blood is very low in oxygen, and it may not be enough to maintain healthy tissues in the body.

Right Ventricular Outflow Tract Obstruction

The third defect in Tetralogy involves an obstruction to blood flow out of the right ventricle. Normally, blood in the right ventricle is pumped into the pulmonary artery toward the lungs for oxygenation. But in this case, there is something blocking the blood's path through the pulmonary artery. Passage of blood may be blocked by bulky muscle tissue in the heart around the opening of the pulmonary valve. Or, sometimes there is a problem with the valve itself. The pulmonary valve opens and closes with each contraction of the ventricle to allow blood to pass into the artery. Sometimes,

FIGURE 9-1
TETRALOGY OF FALLOT

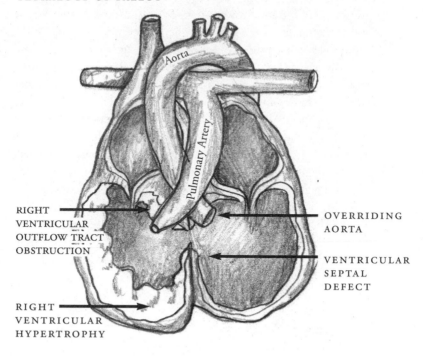

improper formation of the valve may cause the valve to be rigid against the flow of blood.

Right Ventricular Hypertrophy

Because there is a blockage of blood flow to the pulmonary artery, the right ventricle has to work extra hard to get blood flowing to the lungs. As a result, the muscular walls of the right ventricle begin to bulk up. This condition is called Right Ventricular Hypertrophy. The muscle of the ventricle builds up, much like biceps do when they are trained to carry weight. However, the increase in muscle thickness in the heart is not desirable. The enlarged right ventricle pumps very hard in order to eject blood into the pulmonary artery. But, something else also happens. The blood begins to take a new course, the path of least resistance. Instead of going up through the rigid valve (the Right Ventricular Outflow Tract Obstruction), the blood is forcefully ejected across the large defect in the ventricular septal wall. When this happens, deoxygenated blood mixes into oxygenated blood in very large volumes. That blood, which is low in oxygen, is pumped into the aorta toward the body. In turn, the tissues of the body become low in oxygen, and they get cyanotic (blue). This is why a child with Tetralogy of Fallot does not have pink skin and lips. The low oxygen content in the body makes the skin appear pale, dusky, or cyanotic. Cyanosis (blueness) of the skin is a telltale trademark of a child with Tetralogy of Fallot.

Because a large volume of blood in the right ventricle gets shunted to the aorta, there is only a little blood that actually flows into the pulmonary artery. This means that only a small volume of blood will ever even get to the lungs. Consequently, only that small amount of blood gets oxygen exchange. This adds to the cyanosis, and it also adds to the severity of the defect. The more cyanotic the body gets, the harder and faster the heart will work to get oxygen to the tissues. The harder the heart works, the bulkier it becomes. When the heart bulks up, it pumps harder, and more blood shunts through the defects. This creates a vicious cycle that is unproductive and damaging to the heart.

Symptoms to Watch For

Even very small infants who have Tetralogy of Fallot can have symptoms. The amount of the symptoms that they will experience is directly proportional to the amount of obstruction there is to blood flow out of the right ventricle. The more obstruction there is to blood flow going into the pulmonary artery, the more blood crosses over into the left ventricle. Remember, this blood is deoxygenated, and it creates low oxygen concentrations in the blood going to the body. This lowers the body's tissues of oxygen, which can make your child's skin color cyanotic (blue).

Cyanosis

Cyanosis is usually mild at birth and gradually increases as the child gets older. As I explained in the previous section, this is because the muscle of the right ventricle bulks up, causing even more blood to shunt into the aorta. As a result, the child can become even more cyanotic.

Heart Defects in Children

Fatigue

Due to the lack of proper oxygen in the body, your child may become tired very easily. All of the energy the child may have used to laugh, play, and grow is used up by the heart and major organs of the body. In some severe cases, this lack of energy may also interrupt normal feeding patterns and proper weight gain.

Fast Heartbeat and Rapid Breathing

You may notice that your child has a fast heartbeat and rapid breathing. The heart beats fast to help compensate for low oxygen levels in the body. The brain tells the heart to circulate more fresh blood to the tissues, and signals the lungs to make more oxygen available for gas exchange. The child's breathing becomes quick and shallow, and the heart pumps extra fast to circulate this oxygen. This is the body's way of compensating. Unfortunately, the fast heartbeat does not really help in the long run. In fact, after a period of time, the hardworking heart and lungs may add to the child's physical exhaustion.

Clubbing

A condition called "clubbing" of the fingertips and toes can occur as a result of low oxygen levels in the body over a period of approximately six months. Clubbing makes the fingertip look like the finger around the area of the nail has been squashed. The nail bed looks blue or bruised because of low oxygen levels in the blood. Actually, what happens is the tip of the finger grows wider than the last finger joint. It is a very common occurrence in children and adults who have heart defects that cause low oxygen levels in the blood. In time, after the repair of the defect and improved oxygen levels, clubbing of the fingers and toes can slightly improve.

Spells (Squatting)

The most dramatic symptom that your child may experience is unique to children with Tetralogy. It is called a spell, or squatting. Your doctors may ask you about this. If your child's defect is severe, these spells may occur frequently. A spell is caused by periods of extremely low oxygen levels in the body. Some doctors believe the severely low oxygen levels are the result of a spasm in the muscle around the opening of the pulmonary valve (remember, the pulmonary valve opens to allow blood flow to the lungs for oxygen exchange). The muscle surrounding this valve can spasm and close off the opening. When this happens, no blood can get through to the lungs. Consequently, all of the deoxygenated blood in the right ventricle then goes through the VSD into the left ventricle, and it is ejected into the aorta toward the body. Since the lungs during a spell may only receive a trickle of blood flow from the right ventricle, there is only a small amount of oxygen exchange that can take place.

When these spells occur in infants, they may make the lips and nail beds blue, but they can be treated medically with oxygen and rest. However older children can treat themselves. When a spell occurs, the child's immediate reflex is to stop any activity and squat to the floor. The act of squatting increases blood pressures in the upper body, which increases all available blood to flow to the brain and organs. This will temporarily increase oxygen levels in the important areas until the muscle spasm around the pulmonary valve is released. Your doctor will ask you to describe how often your child has spells and what activities bring the spells on. Spells can occur frequently with fevers, warm baths, crying, or physical activity.

Complications Tetralogy of Fallot Can Cause
Heart Pain
Tetralogy of Fallot is a severe defect. It causes children to become cyanotic from low oxygenation. This in itself is a complication of the defect. Also, severely low oxygen levels in the blood can cause heart pain. This is bad because when the heart hurts, it can be from ischemia. Ischemia means that there is not enough oxygen available to meet the needs of the busy heart. Pain from ischemia is the body's way of saying "slow down." But, since the heart cannot slow down, ischemia can cause abnormal heart rhythms.

Clubbing and Shortness of Breath
Older patients with uncorrected Tetralogy can be very sick. They will develop more dramatic clubbing of the fingers and toes. They will experience shortness of breath and intolerance to exercise. More troublesome than these things is a condition that develops called *polycythemia*.

Heart Defects in Children

Polycythemia

Polycythemia means "many cells." The red blood cells in our body carry oxygen. When oxygen levels are low, one way the body tries to compensate for it is to increase the production of red blood cells. The theory is that if there are more red blood cells, then there will be more oxygen. Unfortunately, heart defects that cause cyanosis also cause very low blood oxygen levels, and the body can never really produce enough cells to make the oxygen levels "normal." But, all the brain knows is that the oxygen levels are low, and the body obeys the brain's commands by mass-producing red blood cells. What results are a lot of red blood cells that are immature. Their oxygen-carrying capacity is not even fully developed, and the cells are sticky. This high volume of sticky, immature red blood cells can cause blood clots, strokes, and heart attacks unless treated.

Treatment You Can Expect
Medical Treatment

Medical treatment of Tetralogy of Fallot is aimed directly at preventing and controlling the symptoms and complications—specifically, at raising the oxygen levels in the blood and preventing spells. Your child may need oxygen, medicine, and possibly the transfusion of blood products to treat and prevent the spells. A medication called Inderal is sometimes used to help the heart and its vessels prevent spasms that may lead to spells and low oxygen levels.

In more advanced stages of this illness, polycythemia may develop. This happens as a result of low blood oxygen levels over an extended period of time. With polycythemia, the red blood cells are immature and too abundant. In order to prevent the blood from clotting together and causing strokes or heart attacks, a simple procedure called phlebotomy is performed. In a doctor's office, or perhaps at home with a visiting nurse, blood is removed by a needle. This procedure (sometimes called "bleeding") is done in order to reduce the blood count to safer levels. Phlebotomy may need to be performed at intervals throughout the child's life to keep blood levels safe until the repair of the defect can be performed.

Surgery

Surgical treatment of Tetralogy of Fallot varies. There are a number of factors that will determine which approach your doctor will choose to take. Mostly, these factors include (1) the child's age; (2) the progression of the disease; (3) the degree of symptoms the child is experiencing; and mostly (4) the child's anatomy. Through diagnostic testing (refer to Chapter 13), your doctors can determine if the complete repair of the Tetralogy can be done in one surgery. If the child is healthy, complete repair is the preferred approach. Sometimes, however, the tiny arteries are not fully developed because of months, or years, of low blood flow through them. Low blood flow through the pulmonary artery can make the vessel small and weak. In this case, an initial "palliative" surgery might be needed to redirect some blood flow through the artery. This will prepare the pulmonary artery and tiny lungs for complete repair of the defect in an additional, future surgery (see Figure 9-2).

FIGURE 9-2
A PALLIATIVE SHUNT

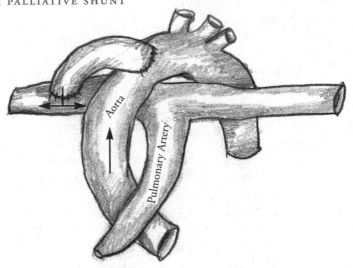

Palliative surgeries (such as "Central Shunts") are done first so that the heart and its vessels are not overloaded when the defect is repaired. Remember, in Tetralogy, most of the blood in the right ventricle is being sent into the aorta. Once the VSD is repaired, all of the blood in the right ventricle will go to the lungs. Neither the pulmonary artery nor the lungs are used to this blood flow. A palliative surgery

Heart Defects in Children

FIGURE 9-3

PLACEMENT OF A VENTRICULAR SEPTAL PATCH

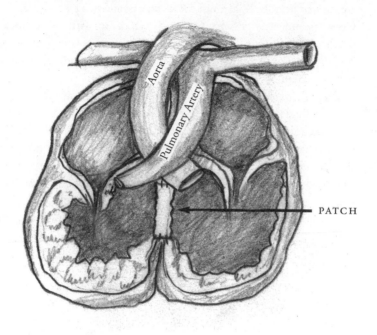

Aorta

Pulmonary Artery

PATCH

will create a shunt for blood to enter the pulmonary artery and lungs in smaller volumes than a complete repair of the defect would. This kind of shunt can prepare the body for normal blood flow that it will receive after the defect is corrected.

If complete repair of the defect is the chosen approach, Tetralogy of Fallot can be repaired in the operating room under anesthesia. After the child is asleep, the surgeon will make an incision down the center of the chest in order to see the heart. The procedure for repairing the Ventricular Septal Defect is the same as described in Chapter 6. A piece of the pericardium, a protective, skinlike sac that covers the heart, can be used to patch up the hole (see Figure 9-3, above). Because it is part of the growing body, this piece of pericardium can be sewn over the hole in the heart. Growing muscle fibers on the septum will mesh with the patch and allow it to grow with the child.

There are also man-made patches that can be used to repair the VSD. These patches are all made of a sterile, sturdy fabric, and they are sutured over the hole much like a knee patch on a pair of trousers. Growing muscle fibers in the heart will mesh with these sterile patches as part of the body's natural healing process. The heart's tissue helps seal the septum and provides a smooth surface where there once was a hole.

Patching of the VSD in Tetralogy of Fallot differs from the patching of a single defect VSD in one important way. The patch placed over the hole in the ventricular septum has to be placed in such a way so that the aorta is separated into the left side of the heart. Remember, in Tetralogy, one of the defects involves the position of the aorta directly over the hole in the septum. This is because as the ventricular septum was developing, it had a slight rotation toward the right side. When the patch is placed over the hole in the septum, it is rotated slightly so that the aorta is enclosed in the left ventricle. Thus, two defects are corrected with one patch: the VSD, and the Overriding Aorta.

Next, the surgeon will correct the resistance to blood flow around the pulmonary artery. In the case where there is bulky muscle tissue under the valve that obstructs blood flow, the surgeon can cut away some of the bulky muscle to remove the obstruction. Sometimes, if there is extensive work to be done to the muscle, another patch can be placed over the area of the valve to widen the valve area. This will allow blood to flow easily to the valve. If the pulmonary valve itself is damaged or undeveloped, it too can be repaired at this time.

The fourth defect, Right Ventricular Hypertrophy, is really a condition that develops as a result of the abnormally large workload of the right ventricle. The bulky muscle of the right ventricle will eventually get smaller as the workload decreases, after the defect is repaired. Just like a bodybuilder's biceps, it will atrophy when it isn't worked out.

What You and Your Child Can Expect in the Future

Today the risks associated with surgical correction of Tetralogy of Fallot vary. The risks of surgery are directly proportional to how sick your child was prior to surgery. The sicker the child, the greater the risk. Your doctor, who knows the exact anatomy and the degree

Heart Defects in Children

of disease within the heart, will be able to explain the risks to you in a personalized way. Usually, the risks of surgery are less than the risks associated with not getting the defects repaired.

Parents who see their sick children immediately after surgical repair and/or palliative surgery are astonished by their children's color. Pink lips, pink fingernails, and pink skin are the most dramatic signs noticeable in those first few hours following surgery. They are an amazingly wonderful sight.

A Special Note to Parents

Your child has no doubt been tired and sick with this defect. I know as a parent that these surgical procedures seem lengthy and frightening. Skilled physicians can correct this defect that has monopolized your child's life and, no doubt, your thoughts. Find the best medical care you can and share your hopes and fears with the team. Remember that no two defects are ever exactly alike. So, try not to compare your child with another who seemingly has the same condition. As always, do not hesitate to communicate directly with your physicians and medical support team regarding your child's unique situation.

Interesting Facts About Tetralogy of Fallot

- Tetralogy of Fallot (Tetralogy) is the most common congenital heart defect in children that causes cyanosis (blueness) of the skin.
- It comprises approximately 9 percent of all congenital heart defects today.
- The first successful surgical treatment of Tetralogy of Fallot was performed in 1945 by Alfred Blalock and Helen Taussig. It was a palliative procedure, their technique is still used today, and the technique is named after them.
- Other defects that may commonly occur with Tetralogy of Fallot include:
    Atrial Septal Defects (ASDs) (Chapter 4);
    Patent Ductus Arteriosus (PDAs) (Chapter 5).

CHAPTER 10

Atrio-Ventricular (A-V) Canal Defect

A-V CANAL IS A difficult defect to understand. Refer frequently to the diagrams, and compare them to the picture of a healthy heart.

An A-V Canal defect is what its name suggests: a defect (canal) between the atria and the ventricles. As we discussed in Chapter 2, "The Healthy Heart," the atria are the two top chambers of the heart. The right atrium collects deoxygenated blood coming from the body. The left atrium collects oxygenated blood from the lungs. Blood is then passed through the tricuspid valve on the right side, and the mitral valve on the left side, into the ventricles. The ventricles are the two bottom chambers of the heart. They are responsible for forcefully pumping blood out of the heart. Blood is pumped to the lungs for oxygen from the right side, and to the body to provide energy from the left side. The right and left sides of the heart work together and form the "lub-dub" sounds of your heartbeat.

In A-V Canal there are defects in the septums (walls) inside the heart. The septums are muscular walls that divide the four chambers of the heart: the two atria and the two ventricles. Without a septum dividing the chambers into four, the heart would look like a hollow ball.

During development of the heart in utero, the septal walls grow from the outside-in. When development is complete, the four walls meet in the middle of the heart and join to form the four totally separate chambers. An A-V Canal defect is the result of misalignment of the septal walls, or improper formation of the chambers.

Three Degrees of Severity

There are different degrees of severity of an A-V Canal defect. They can generally be grouped into three different categories in order of least serious to most serious: Partial, Intermediate, and Complete.

Partial A-V Canal

Partial A-V Canal is the least serious of the three variations. This defect is the combination of an atrial Septal Defect (see Chapter 4) and a Ventricular Septal Defect (see Chapter 6). In Partial A-V Canal, these two defects occur together, and they occur near each other. In other words, the defect in the atrial septum is low on the septal wall, and the defect in the ventricular septum is high on the septal wall. The close proximity of the defects usually cause a problem with one of the valves in the heart. The mitral valve, which separates the left atrium and the left ventricle on the left side of the heart, may develop very slightly deformed. Because of this deformity, over time the valve can become damaged from blood flow through it.

Intermediate A-V Canal

The intermediate form of A-V Canal is more serious. In this case, the septums that grow in toward each other during development do not actually meet. As the heart pumps, there is no real division of the chambers. Instead of four separate chambers, there is one large one. When the heart pumps, blood leaks through the hole in the septum and mixes abnormally in all four chambers. The valves that usually separate the atria and ventricles are sometimes defective too. The mitral valve on the left side of the heart is almost always deformed. The center part of the valve that opens and closes with blood flow is usually not functioning properly. As a result, blood is constantly leaking through the valve abnormally.

Complete A-V Canal

The complete form of A-V Canal is the most serious. It is similar to Partial A-V Canal in that the septum does not meet in the center of the heart (see Figure 10-1). There is a very large hollow hole between the four chambers. As the heart pumps, blood is ejected everywhere, in no specific direction. There is no differentiation of oxygenated and deoxygenated blood. It is all mixed, in one large chamber, being pumped everywhere. Try to visualize a heart with complete A-V canal

FIGURE 10-1

COMPLETE ATRIO-VENTRICULAR CANAL DEFECT

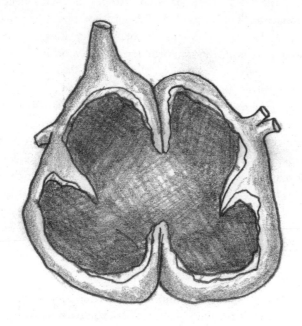

as a hollow ball. If you put oxygenated blood in on one side, and nonoxygenated blood on another side, and then squeeze it, there is no way to keep the blood separate. All of the blood will mix, and in the heart there is no way to send nonoxygenated blood to the lungs and oxygenated blood to the body. The mixed blood that is sent to the lungs is abnormally high in oxygen, and the blood going to the body is abnormally low in oxygen.

The two valves that normally separate the upper atria from the lower ventricles are deformed too. Because there is no septum in the center of the heart for the valves to "anchor" onto, the valves grow together. Instead of being separate, the tricuspid and mitral valves fuse and form one common valve. This complicates the blood flow even more.

As we have discussed, blood flow through the heart is very specific. In the case of complete a-v Canal, there is pandemonium and chaos in the direction of the blood flow.

Symptoms to Watch For

The amount of symptoms your child may have will depend on the severity of the defect. Some children with partial A-V Canal defects may not have any symptoms. Children with complete A-V Canal defects usually have severe symptoms before they are one year old. Some even have symptoms before they are one month old.

Lung Infections and Cyanosis

There are many common symptoms that occur as a result of this defect. Children may experience frequent infections in the lungs, including colds, and may even develop cyanosis (blueness) of the skin. In this case, cyanosis occurs because freshly oxygenated blood on the left side of the heart is mixed with deoxygenated blood from the right side. This lowers the concentration of oxygen in the blood stream, and the body does not get enough oxygen in the tissues and muscles. Low oxygen levels in the tissues of the body can cause blueness of the skin, lips, and fingertips.

Fatigue

Due to the lack of oxygen in the body, the child may become tired very easily. All of the energy your child may have used to laugh, play, and grow is used up by the heart and major organs of the body because they are deprived of sufficient oxygen. In more severe cases, this lack of energy may also interrupt normal feeding habits and prevent normal weight gain.

Fast Heartbeat and Rapid Breathing

You may notice that your child has a fast heartbeat and rapid breathing. The heart beats fast to help compensate for low oxygen levels in the body. The brain tells the heart to circulate more fresh blood to the tissues and signals the lungs to make more oxygen available for gas exchange. As a result, the child's breathing becomes quick and shallow to get more oxygen in the lungs, and the heart pumps extra fast to circulate the oxygen. This is the body's way of compensating. Unfortunately, these compensatory mechanisms do not really help in the long run. In fact, after a period of time, the hardworking heart and lungs can add to the child's physical exhaustion.

Clubbing

A condition called "clubbing" of the fingertips and toes can occur as a result of low oxygen levels in the body over a period of approximately six months. Clubbing makes the fingertip look like it has been squashed. The nail bed looks blue or bruised because of low oxygen levels in the blood. Actually, what happens is the tip of the finger grows wider than the last finger joint. It is a very common occurrence in children and adults who have heart defects that cause low oxygen levels in the blood. In time, after the repair of the defect, improved oxygen levels in the blood can slightly improve this clubbing of the fingers and toes.

Complications A-V Canal Can Cause

Complete A-V Canal is a very serious heart defect. An estimated 90 percent of children with this defect will develop severe lung disease from the chaotic flow of blood. Severe lung disease may even develop before the child is one year old. Once the irreversible lung disease occurs, there is an associated high mortality rate. This is why early treatment is imperative, and complete surgical repair should be performed as soon as possible.

Treatment You Can Expect

Medical treatment of A-V Canal is aimed directly at preventing and controlling symptoms and complications of the defect—specifically, at raising the oxygen levels in the blood and preventing respiratory infections. In the hospital, prior to surgery, special measures may be taken to promote nutrition and growth. Feeding tubes may be used to give the child nourishment. The primary goal will be to keep your child healthy until surgical correction of the defect can be performed.

Surgery

All children, even young babies, are given total anesthesia so that they are asleep through the entire operation. Once the child is under anesthesia, A-V Canal can be repaired in the operating room. After the child is asleep, the surgeon will make an incision down the center of the chest in order to see the heart. For all three variations of A-V Canal, there is one basic approach to surgically correcting the defect. First, the Atrial Septal Defect is repaired. Second, the

Ventricular Septal Defect is repaired. Then, the two valves that divide the atria and ventricles (the tricuspid valve on the right and the mitral valve on the left) are repaired. Remember, no two children with the same defect are exactly the same. The extent to which reconstruction of the heart is needed will vary with each child.

To repair the atrial and ventricular septums, a sterile patch made of durable fabric is sutured into the heart where the septum should be. These sterile patches are sewn in such a way that four separate chambers are created. Growing muscle fibers in the heart will eventually mesh with these patches as part of the body's natural healing process. The heart's tissue will help seal the septum and provide a smooth surface where there once was a defect.

Next, the tricuspid valve, between the right atrium and the right ventricle, is inspected and corrected. If there is a problem with blood flow through it, it can be repaired. Sometimes, all the valve may need is to have the opening clipped a little so it is not rigid to blood flow. In other cases, however, as in the case of complete A-V Canal, there may not even be a separate valve for the right side of the heart. In this case, more extensive surgery is performed to create a valve at that site.

Last, the mitral valve, between the left atrium and left ventricle, is inspected and repaired. There is almost always damage to this valve, and usually there are developmental defects involved in the structure of the valve. Extensive reconstruction of this valve is almost always involved as part of the repair process of complete A-V Canal. Because all children have a different anatomy, and no two with the same defects are ever exactly the same, your surgeon can explain to you what exactly will be needed to repair the valves in your child's heart.

What You and Your Child Can Expect in the Future

The risks associated with surgical correction of A-V Canal vary immensely. Surgical risk is directly proportional to how sick your child is. The sicker the child is prior to surgery, the greater the risk is. Your doctor, who knows the exact anatomy and the degree of reconstruction needed in your child's heart, will be able to explain the risks to you in a personalized way. Usually the risks of surgery are less than the risks associated with not getting the defect repaired.

Parents who see their sick children immediately after surgical repair of this defect are astonished by their children's color. Pink lips, pink fingernails, and pink skin are the most dramatic signs noticeable in those first few hours following surgery. They are an amazingly wonderful sight.

In some cases, the need for another surgery (after the initial correction) arises. This is usually because of the valves. Children who need total reconstruction of their tricuspid and mitral valves may develop a small amount of leaking blood through them. Sometimes this sounds more serious than it actually is, but in other cases, the valve might need additional repair. Another reason for a second operation usually involves the ventricular septum. Because the ventricles pump so forcefully, blood pressure against the sterile patch is high. This can cause small leaks through the patched areas and, especially, at the area of the sutures.

A Special Note to Parents

A-v Canal is a serious defect. Your child has no doubt been tired and sick. I know as a parent that these surgical procedures seem lengthy and frightening. Skilled physicians can correct this defect that has monopolized your lives. Find the best possible medical and surgical care you can, and place your hopes and fears in their hands. No two defects are ever exactly alike, so try not to compare your child with another who seemingly has the same condition. As always, do not hesitate to communicate directly with your physicians and medical support team regarding your child's unique situation.

Interesting Facts About A-V Canal

- A-v Canal defects account for approximately 4 percent of all congenital heart defects.
- A-v Canal defects represent between 30 to 40 percent of all heart defects seen in children with Down's syndrome.
- The first successful repair of a complete A-v Canal defect was performed in 1955 by Dr. Lillehei and colleagues.

CHAPTER 11

Other Heart Defects

THERE ARE SO MANY congenital defects that it is not possible to cover them all in this book. I created this chapter to make sure that your child's defect is not missed. Sit down with your child's physicians and medical support team. Let them help you fill out the worksheet provided on page 105. Write in your book, draw in your book, and personalize it for your child's own unique situation.

Some of the defects you may be experiencing are listed below.

Anomalous Pulmonary Venous Drainage
This condition is characterized by abnormal positioning of the veins that drain blood into the heart. The two main vessels that are involved in this defect are the inferior and superior vena cavas. These veins bring deoxygenated blood back to the heart from the body. Normally, they should be connected to the right atrium. Often, they can be misaligned, or connected to other structures around the heart. If they eventually drain into the right atrium, there may not be a problem. If, however, these veins are connected to the left atrium, they are bringing deoxygenated blood to the left side of the heart, which is going to send that blood back to the body and not to the lungs. In this case, surgery may be needed to redirect the blood back into the right side of the heart.

Double Outlet Left Ventricle
In this defect, there is usually a very large hole in the wall between the right and left ventricles (the ventricular septum). Sometimes the ventricular septum is absent. Refer to Chapter 6, "Ventricular Septal Defects (VSDs)." The pulmonary artery, which is supposed to

be on the right side of the heart, can gain access to the left ventricle through the hole in the ventricular septum. Double Outlet Left Ventricle is diagnosed in a child when the left ventricle supplies most of the blood to both the aorta and the pulmonary artery.

Double Outlet Right Ventricle

This defect is very similar to Tetralogy of Fallot. Refer to Chapter 9 for a detailed explanation of these defects. Double Outlet Right Ventricle is diagnosed in a child with Tetralogy of Fallot if 90 percent of the aorta is coming from the right ventricle.

Hypoplastic Left Heart Syndrome

This is a very serious congenital heart defect. It is characterized by the severe underdevelopment of the left ventricle. The left ventricle is the "workhorse" of the heart. It is responsible for pumping freshly oxygenated blood to all areas of the body. In a severe Hypoplastic Left Heart Syndrome, the left ventricle is too small and too weak to adequately circulate blood to the body. In some children, surgery is needed to help sustain life very shortly after the diagnosis of this defect.

Pulmonary Atresia

This is a very serious congenital heart defect. Atresia is the absence of a normal opening or canal. In Pulmonary Atresia, there is usually a profound underdevelopment, or even absence, of the pulmonary artery and/or the pulmonary valve. The pulmonary artery collects blood from the right ventricle in the heart and sends it to the lungs to be oxygenated. If blood cannot enter the artery, it cannot get to the lungs. Often there are other defects present in the heart to help redirect blood flow to the lungs. Two such defects are Atrial Septal Defects (Chapter 4) and Patent Ductus Arteriosus (Chapter 5). Surgery is most often needed to help reconstruct the pulmonary artery and to increase blood flow to the lungs.

Pulmonary Stenosis

The pulmonary artery is the large vessel that brings deoxygenated blood from the right ventricle in the heart to the lungs. *Stenosis* is a term used to describe a stricture on the pulmonary artery, or a problem with the pulmonary valve, which causes resistance to blood flow through the artery. If blood has trouble getting through the pulmonary artery, then the amount of blood that can get to the lungs for oxygen is limited. Some examples of Pulmonary Stenosis can be found in Chapter 9, "Tetralogy of Fallot."

Transposition of the Great Vessels

In this defect, the two greatest vessels in the body, the pulmonary artery and the aorta, are transposed. This means that the aorta and pulmonary artery are switched. Instead of the aorta coming from the left ventricle, it comes from the right ventricle. And, instead of the pulmonary artery coming from the right ventricle, it comes from the left ventricle. This sounds simple, but it can actually become confusing because the heart may switch development of the ventricles. That means that there may be switched development of the inner lining and muscle mass within the ventricles. This changes the predictability of the force of contractions from the right ventricle (which should be weaker), and the left ventricle (which should be stronger).

Tricuspid Atresia

This is a very serious congenital heart defect. Atresia is the absence of a normal opening or canal. Tricuspid Atresia describes the absence, or closure, of the tricuspid valve. As we discussed in Chapter 2, "The Healthy Heart," the tricuspid valve allows blood to pass from the right atrium into the right ventricle. From there, deoxygenated blood is sent toward the lungs to get oxygenated. When there is no tricuspid valve, blood cannot enter the right ventricle or get to the lungs for oxygen. This defect is potentially life-threatening unless there is another defect associated with it that allows blood to enter the lungs. Often, two other defects that are associated with maintaining blood flow to the lungs in tricuspid atresia are Patent Ductus Arteriosus (Chapter 5) and Atrial Septal Defects (Chapter 4).

Truncus Arteriosus

This defect describes the incomplete development of the aorta and the pulmonary artery. During the formation of the heart and its vessels in utero, the pulmonary artery and aorta begin as one large "trunk" of an artery. Eventually, as the heart twists and out-patches, the aorta and the pulmonary artery separate to form two distinctly separate vessels. In Truncus Arteriosus, the complete separation of these two vessels fails to occur. The arterial trunk usually ends up being positioned over a large hole in the wall between the right and left ventricle (see "Ventricular Septal Defects," Chapter 6).

Vascular Rings

Vascular Rings describe a condition that occurs as the result of abnormal development of the aortic arch. The aorta is the largest artery in the body. It brings freshly oxygenated blood from the left ventricle in the heart to all organs and tissues of the body. The aortic arch is the area on the aorta where it reaches up out of the heart and arches around to go back down toward the body. Abnormal development of the arch can cause compression of or around the windpipe (trachea), or the esophagus. The aorta, or the arteries coming from the aorta, can actually develop in a ring around these structures, and strangle them. Surgery can be done to alleviate this pressure and to redirect the arteries.

A Special Note to Parents

Always remember that no two defects are ever exactly alike. If there is another child that you know who has the "same" defect as your child, don't be fooled. Every child acts and reacts differently to medical and surgical treatment. There are so many factors that influence the recovery of children with congenital heart defects.

Your child has, no doubt, been sick and tired with this heart disease. I know as a parent that medical and surgical procedures can seem lengthy and frightening. Find the best medical and surgical care you can. As always, do not hesitate to speak with your physicians and medical support team regarding your child's own unique situation.

Our Defect _____

Explanation:
- What is it?
- What does it look like?
- How did it happen?

Symptoms:
- What symptoms should I look for?
- What symptoms should I expect?

Complications:
- Are there any serious complications of this defect if it is not repaired?

Medical Treatment:
- Is there any medical treatment for this defect?
- Is there any medicine that will help my child feel better?

Surgical Treatment:
A lot of the defects in this section may require more than one surgery to be repaired. Sometimes, because of the way that the heart and lungs develop, preliminary surgery must be performed. Be sure to discuss this with your doctor.

- Is there any surgical treatment?
- Is surgery a cure?
- Will one operation fix it, or should we expect the need for any additional surgery?
- What exactly is done in surgery to repair the defect?

Expectations:
- What expectations should we have for the future health of our child?

Part Three
What You Must Know

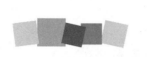

CHAPTER 12

Infection of the Heart and Its Valves

Bacterial Endocarditis

Infection in the heart is a very serious condition that develops in many children who have congenital heart defects. It is very important that you know about this condition, and learn to recognize its symptoms, so that you can protect your child from it.

You may already know that many different forms of bacteria live on and in our bodies. Our mouth, stomach, and intestines are home to a large amount of bacteria. The surface of our skin also carries a lot of bacteria that we cannot see, and they do not cause us any harm. However, the blood in our body is sterile. There is absolutely no bacteria in it at all. If bacteria do enter the bloodstream, they can grow and cause infection. Infections that grow in the heart are called Bacterial Endocarditis.

When bacteria get into the bloodstream of any person with a congenital heart defect, the bacteria tend to be attracted to the heart because bacteria are attracted to turbulent blood flow. Since turbulent blood flow is created by certain heart defects, a heart defect—or an implanted structure in the heart—that prevents blood flow from being smooth and natural can attract bacteria. What usually happens is that the bacteria begins to collect on the heart's valves, or on any structure in the heart.

Endocarditis means swelling, or inflammation, of the heart tissue. When this inflammation is caused by bacteria (bacterial endocarditis), it is especially dangerous because it can cause a substantial amount of damage to the heart and its valves. Before the invention of antibiotics these infections were almost certainly fatal. However, with antibiotics, and other medications that can decrease inflammation in the heart, we can fight, treat, and cure these infections rather quickly. But early diagnosis and quick treatment of Bacterial Endocarditis is essential.

Children who have a defect that is not yet corrected run a higher risk of developing Bacterial Endocarditis than a child with a corrected defect. This is because of turbulent blood flow around the area of the defect. Generally, once the heart is repaired, the risk of contracting these infections will decrease, but it is not completely eliminated. This is very important to understand, because some children who have had their heart defects fixed will grow normally to adulthood but still need to be continually cautious of these infections.

Symptoms to Watch For

Infections cause fevers. Sometimes, a fever will be the first sign that your child has an infection. In fact, if your child has a congenital heart defect and develops a prolonged fever that does not have an obvious cause, you should suspect that it is from Bacterial Endocarditis, and you should call your doctor right away. Likewise, if the child has been sick with another kind of infection (ear infection, etc.) and continues to run a fever that does not subside after medical treatment, be suspicious that the infection may have spread to the heart and call your doctor.

Other symptoms your child may have that could be associated with an infection in the body and indicate that Bacterial Endocarditis might be present include:

- physical exhaustion or fatigue;
- a sudden decrease in appetite or a low desire to eat;
- achy or painful muscles, or joints without an obvious injury;
- prolonged headaches; and
- uncharacteristic irritability in an otherwise easygoing infant or child.

Since your child has had a defect in the structure of the heart, your doctor will frequently examine your child to listen for any changes in the sound of the heartbeat. A murmur is a sound that the heart makes when there is turbulent blood flow in the heart. Some kids with congenital heart defects have murmurs even after their heart defect has been repaired, and this is normal. However, if your doctor suspects Bacterial Endocarditis and hears a change in your child's murmur, it may mean that the infection is causing damage to the valves in the heart. Or, if a murmur shows up in a child who did not previously have one, an infection could have caused the valves in the heart to become ineffective, and a murmur could be the first sign that something is wrong.

How to Diagnose Bacterial Endocarditis

If an infection develops in or around the heart, bacteria will be found in the blood. There are many different kinds of bacteria that cause infections in the heart. In order to find this bacteria, a sample of blood from your child will be drawn and sent to a clinical laboratory to be cultured. In the lab, technicians can run tests to see which antibiotic will be most successful in treating the infection. If bacteria is found in your child's blood sample, your doctor will prescribe the best antibiotic for the infection.

Medical Treatment of Bacterial Endocarditis
Antibiotics

Once your child has been diagnosed with bacterial endocarditis, the child must be started on antibiotics. What kind of antibiotic is prescribed, and how long it should be taken, will depend on the kind of bacteria that is found in the blood. Some resistant kinds of bacteria may require more aggressive treatment than others. Six weeks or more of antibiotic therapy is common to stop some infections. It is essential that you finish all medications that are prescribed, even if it seems that your child is better. Bacteria that may still be alive in your child's body can get used to living in the presence of the antibiotics and become resistant to them. So, unless your doctor says otherwise, finish the entire prescription. If you do not, resistant bacteria can flourish and grow even stronger.

When your child completes the regimen of antibiotics and is well again, additional blood cultures should be done to ensure that the infection is totally gone. Some physicians will check blood cultures several times in the two to three months that follow an infection to make sure that it does not reoccur.

Surgery

If an infection from Bacterial Endocarditis is very severe, it can damage the heart to the point that it requires surgery to repair it. Or, sometimes surgery is required to scrape off infected areas of the heart that antibiotics cannot eradicate. Surgery is also required if the bacterial infections have formed abscesses or pockets of infection in the heart that need to be removed. If your child develops Bacterial Endocarditis while waiting to electively repair the heart defect, antibiotics will be used to clear the infection. Once the child is well again, surgery to correct the heart defect should not be postponed. Once children have had Bacterial Endocarditis, they are at a higher risk of contracting it again. Repair of the heart defect will, in most cases, decrease the risk of redeveloping the infection.

How to Prevent Bacterial Endocarditis

Bacterial endocarditis can occur in a person of any age, with any congenital heart defect. However, it is most frequently found in children with the following five defects:
- Patent Ductus Arteriosus (Chapter 5);
- Ventricular Septal Defects (Chapter 6);
- Aortic Stenosis (Chapter 7);
- Coarctation of the Aorta (Chapter 8); and
- Tetralogy of Fallot (Chapter 9).

To prevent the onset of an infection, some children will need to receive antibiotics prior to any invasive medical procedure for the rest of their lives, especially if they have one of the five common defects listed here. But, infections are not selective; they can occur in any child with a heart defect. As always, speak with your doctor about the need for antibiotics prior to your child having any of the following procedures, and be alert for the signs and symptoms of an infection. (And remember, these concerns will follow your child into and throughout adulthood.)

Antibiotics may be necessary prior to surgery, or any invasive procedure such as:

DENTAL PROCEDURES. This includes routine cleanings. Bacterial Endocarditis associated with dental work occurs frequently. This is mostly due to the high amount of bacteria normally found in the mouth. Anything that can make your child's gums bleed, even aggressive tooth brushing, can give the bacteria a way to enter the bloodstream and cause infection.

MOST SURGICAL PROCEDURES. This especially includes the following:
- Tonsillectomy;
- Bronchoscopy;
- Vaginal Hysterectomy;
- Vaginal Childbirth (if there is an infection present);
- Any abdominal surgery;
- Any bladder surgery, which also includes cystoscopies and procedures done to widen the tubes leading to the bladder. This also includes the placement of a urinary catheter if there is a urinary tract infection present.

OTHER PROCEDURES. This includes the following:
- Respiratory Tract (lungs);
- Gastrointestinal Tract (mouth to intestines);
- Urinary Tract (bladder and kidneys);
- Reproductive Tract.

If your child is at a high risk of contracting a heart infection and has any prolonged fever (even if it is from something that has been diagnosed, such as pneumonia or a urinary tract infection), the child can still develop Bacterial Endocarditis. Bacteria in the body can migrate from one place to another via the blood supply, and may end up infecting the heart.

You must become aware, and wary, of Bacterial Endocarditis, and teach your child to consciously prevent it as the child grows to adulthood. It is paramount to your child's continued good health.

CHAPTER 13

Common Tests Your Child May Need

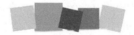

THERE ARE A NUMBER of tests that your child may have to undergo in order to diagnose and treat a heart defect. I designed this chapter to help you understand these tests and prepare your child for them. Mostly, tests are run to give physicians the most accurate picture possible of your child's defect. Different tests will give different information about the location and severity of a defect. Common tests that will be run on your child can be found in this chapter.

Chest X-Ray

A chest x-ray can be done at intervals during your child's illness. This test can give the doctor information on the size of the heart and the status of the child's lungs. Very often, a troubled heart will cause abnormal fluid accumulation in the body, and especially the lungs. X-rays can be performed at any time of the day. Your child does not need to be fasting or taking any special medication in order to be able to have this test. X-rays can be developed in minutes and will provide the doctors with important information, sometimes while you are still waiting in the office.

An x-ray done today can be compared to one that was done months, even years, ago to determine if there is any progression of the heart's failure. If the picture of your child's lungs and heart from an x-ray worsens, your physician may prescribe any one of the following tests.

Echocardiogram

An echocardiogram is a procedure for studying the structure and motion of the heart. It is not an invasive procedure, and it is not uncomfortable. This test uses sound waves (ultrasound) that bounce off the heart to create a picture on a screen. The picture from an echocardiogram can trace blood flow through the heart. By watching the blood flow, abnormalities can be found in the structure of the heart and its valves. The picture that is obtained from an echocardiogram is probably the best tool physicians have of viewing the heart in a noninvasive way.

There are no preliminary measures that need to be done prior to an echocardiogram. Like the x-ray, this test does not require that the child fast or take any special medications in order to have this test performed. Your child will need to lie flat on the back. The chest area will be exposed, and a clear jell will be smeared across it. The jell helps the ultrasound to transmit a picture to the machine at the side of the bed. Usually, an ultrasound only takes about fifteen minutes to complete. The results are recorded on a videotape so that your doctor can review the film several times. If your doctor performs the procedure, he or she may be able to give you the results immediately as the pictures are being provided by the ultrasound.

Electrocardiogram (EKG)

An EKG is a test used to show the electrical tracing of the heartbeat. Sticky pads, which sense the electrical impulses from the heart, are placed on the chest in specific locations. These pads transmit impulses to a machine that draws the tracing of the heartbeat. EKGs provide information about the electrical activity of the heart. If the heart is enlarged as a result of a defect, an EKG will show that as well.

EKGs are done to ensure that the heart is beating regularly. If the heart beats too slow, too fast, or irregularly, the EKG will trace its activity. With this information, the doctor may be able to adjust any medications your child may be on. EKGs are used in conjunction with other tests mentioned in this chapter, and for monitoring purposes after surgery.

Cardiac Catheterization

A cardiac catheterization is the most sophisticated tool the doctor has for making a diagnosis of your child's heart defect. It is an invasive procedure that is done in a hospital by a physician. As its name suggests, a cardiac catheterization requires a tube (catheter) to be passed into the heart. This is done by inserting a tube into an

Heart Defects in Children

artery or vein in the child's arm or leg. When the catheter reaches the area that the doctor wishes to see, a dye may be injected into the heart through the catheter. Moving pictures can then be taken of the heart by a special machine above the bed. Moving pictures of blood flow will show the doctor if there are any defects in the child's heart or valves. These pictures can be unbelievably clear and precise. The pictures are recorded on videotapes, and if your child requires any surgical intervention, they can guide the doctors to the exact location in the heart that is causing a problem. The videotapes help to eliminate extra time in the operating room looking for defects. It also helps minimize the possibility that the surgeon might find a second, hidden defect in the operating room that is unexpected.

Preparation for a cardiac catheterization is almost the same as for having an operation. On the night before the procedure, your child may be required to take a bath with a special antiseptic soap (Betadine). The soap is reddish brown and may look yucky to the child. Be sure to rinse the child thoroughly. It is very important that your child have an empty stomach prior to the procedure to prevent vomiting during the study. You will get instructions to stop all food and water after a certain time at night or in the morning.

Prior to the procedure, a doctor or nurse will give the child medicine to induce sleep. Most children will be asleep for the entire procedure. The actual time that your child will be in the catheterization lab will depend on how complex the heart defect is. Usually though, the entire study lasts between one and two hours.

Nearly all children go home the day of, or the day after, the procedure unless they have been previously scheduled for surgery during the same hospital admission. In most cases your child may return to school on the next day, unless your doctor advises against it. Do not allow the catheterization site (where the tube was inserted) to get wet until it scabs (about two to three days). Change the bandage daily, whenever it gets wet, or with each diaper change (if your child is still in diapers). Once there is a scab, the bandage may be removed.

If you notice any drainage or redness around the catheterization site, notify your doctor immediately. If there are stitches at the area of the catheterization site, contact your doctor for a date that the stitches should be removed. This is usually done one week to ten days after the procedure.

Magnetic Resonance Imaging (MRIs)

An MRI might be performed on your child to evaluate a structural defect on the outside of the heart. These kinds of defects would involve problems with the major vessels surrounding the heart. An MRI is a test done with a huge magnet. It does not hurt, and it is not invasive. The picture an MRI provides for doctors is an accurate, sharp picture of all of the structures in the chest, and their proximity to the heart.

For an MRI, the child must be able to lie flat on the back for a period of about twenty minutes. The machine can be very loud and scary, but it does not touch or hurt. The child is placed inside a large, hollow tube in the machine, which can be frightening for young children. But because it is not invasive, it is sometimes a more acceptable test for parents. Unfortunately, MRIs are not commonly used for the diagnosis of heart defects, and they can be expensive.

Blood Tests and Urine Tests

Blood and urine tests are usually done prior to surgery. The urine is tested to make sure there is no infection. If any infection is found, invasive procedures may be postponed until antibiotics can correct it. Blood tests are done to check for a variety of things. A complete blood count can alert the doctors to any infection in the body. A hemoglobin and hematocrit test will be done to make sure that those levels are in a safe range for surgery. Also tested are electrolytes, and blood sugar levels. If these tests are off at all, the levels can be corrected with medication.

CHAPTER 14

If Your Child Needs Surgery

SOMETIMES SURGERY IS the only answer for a congenital heart defect. It is always frightening. I designed this chapter to help you be able to anticipate what will happen around the surgery. I hope that it will serve to alleviate some fears, and to better equip you and your child emotionally for what lies ahead.

At least two weeks prior to surgery, you might want to check with your hospital about options for donating blood to be used for your child. This is called "directed donor" blood. If your child should need a transfusion during or after surgery, the child will get the blood that you donated instead of blood from the general population. There are very good tests being used today to screen blood both from the general population and from directed donors. Directed donor blood is simply an option you may choose, to alleviate additional concern around the operation.

Preparing Your Child for Surgery

To prepare your child emotionally for surgery, you are the judge. Depending on your child's age and level of maturity, there are many ways to approach this. You know your child best. If you are unsure, libraries contain many books on children and their developmental stages. These books can help you put things into simple terminology and teach you how to explain things like this to your children. Some hospitals give out simple children's literature or coloring books explaining what will happen. Be sure to use every resource available to you.

In most cases, your child will be admitted to the hospital on the day before, or the day of, the surgery. Either way, there are some pre-operative tests that will need to be done before surgery. They will most likely include blood tests, urine tests, a chest x-ray, and an electrocardiogram (EKG). Please refer to Chapter 13 for a more detailed explanation about these tests. In some hospitals, you may be able to get an advance tour of the intensive care unit (ICU) that your child will be in after surgery. You should expect a visit from the surgical team before the surgery, and also from an anesthesiologist. There will be several consents that you will be asked to sign for the surgery, anesthesia, and possibility of blood administration. This is all likely to be stressful. If you are a single parent, you may want to ask a friend or relative to join you for support. Be sure that all of your questions are answered satisfactorily by your medical support team prior to surgery. (Please refer to Chapter 15 for a list of some questions you may need to ask your doctors.)

The night before surgery your child may have to bathe with an antiseptic soap (Betadine). This is done to eliminate germs and to decrease the amount of normal bacteria that lives on the skin. The nursing staff may be able to show you and your child pictures that will give you an idea of what to expect while your child is in the intensive care unit. In most cases, your child will not be able to eat or drink anything after midnight. For this reason, you may want to encourage a late-night snack before bedtime.

The Day of the Surgery

Depending on what time your child is scheduled to go to the operating room, this morning can be a tough one. Young children especially have a hard time understanding why they are not allowed to eat when they are hungry. Some small children may need to be on intravenous fluids so that their blood sugars do not get too low in the morning. Before your child is taken to surgery, the child will be given a sedative to relax, and, possibly, to sleep.

During surgery, most hospitals will direct you to a place where you can wait. Your doctor will give you an idea of approximately how long the operation will take. Once the operation is done, someone from the surgical team will usually meet you in the waiting area to let you know how everything is. Don't be alarmed if the surgery takes longer than expected. Normal delays are common, and they usually do not have anything to do with your child's condition. If you think you have been waiting too long, the pediatric unit should

Heart Defects in Children

be able to furnish you with a number you can call to check on the status of the operation.

After the Surgery

Immediately following the surgery, your child will be taken to the recovery area for open heart surgery. Sometimes, this is in the ICU. In this area your child will be under constant observation with monitoring systems. The amount of time your child will have to spend in the ICU depends on what kind of surgery was performed. Remember, no two children with the same defect will react the same way.

Visiting hours vary from hospital to hospital. When you speak with the doctor after surgery, be sure to ask when you will be permitted to see your child. In some institutions, you will be able to stay a while with your child immediately following the surgery. Chances are, your child will be asleep. Once you know that the child is OK, this might be a good time for you to get something to eat and take care of you. Moms and dads become in big demand over the next few days, and you will need to be rested.

There are many things that you should be prepared to see right after surgery. There will be many tubes and wires hooked up to your child. Each one has a specific, and important, function. Little by little, as the days in ICU progress, these tubes will be eliminated when they are not needed. Try, if you can, to see past these horrible tubes and to focus on your baby. Children are magicians at picking up stress from their parents, and your worried eyes may frighten them. Most important, do not be afraid to touch and kiss your child, which is reassuring. If your child has a special toy or blanket (like my son has), be sure to bring it to the ICU. It will be very comforting for your child to have a familiar object as the child wakes up.

Pain Control

The medications used during anesthesia can last throughout the night. They not only make your child sleepy, they also help to control pain. Once these medications wear off, your child will receive medication as necessary to alleviate pain. The dosage of medication is calculated to the child's body weight. It is very specific, and it is usually very effective.

It will be uncomfortable in the days ahead for your child to move and cough. Moving and coughing are a very important part of recovery, and despite the hurt, it is important that you encourage your child to do the prescribed activities. However, being uncomfortable and being in pain are two different things. Work closely with your medical support team, and speak for your child when you need to. Pain medication will usually not come automatically; you may need to ask for it.

Recovery in the Hospital

As the days progress and the tubes are discontinued, the medical staff will gradually increase your child's activity. They will continue to check your child's temperature, heart rate, and blood pressure at intervals throughout the day. Your child may also be weighed daily to assess the amount of water retention following surgery. There will be play therapy and special exercises to do.

It may be important in the hospital to record any food or fluid intake that your child may have, and to keep a record of urine output. Sometimes, fluid restrictions are necessary if the child has more fluid intake than output. Fluid restrictions can be frustrating for the child, who may not understand them. These times can be trying for you as well. Patience and firm guidance is necessary, along with a lot of love.

Recovery at Home

Medications are a big part of recovery at home. You must know how to give them, and you must watch for their possible side effects. It is important that you know what times they should be administered, and what they do. The nursing staff in the hospital should be able to give you all of the information you will need. Be sure to keep medication information handy so you can refer to it frequently. (A list of some commonly used medications is included in pages 137 through 139 of this book.)

If it is OK with your doctor, once the incision has a scab on it, your child may bathe in a tub or shower. Be sure to clean the incision and other wounds with soap and water unless your doctor directs you otherwise. It is important to protect the incision from sunburn, and to dress your child in soft clothing as the incision heals. It may be sensitive for a while even after it has healed. If you notice any redness, swelling, or leakage from any incision or wound be sure to contact your doctor immediately. Any of those symptoms can be a sign that there is an underlying infection that may need to be treated immediately.

After surgery, be sure to postpone your child's dental work and immunizations for at least three months. Dental work should only be done before three months if it is absolutely necessary, and if it is OK with your cardiologist. Be sure that you tell your dentist about the surgery. Your child should be on antibiotics before any dental work is done. Antibiotics are used to prevent infections that may lead to Bacterial Endocarditis. (Refer to Chapter 12 for an explanation of this infection in the heart.)

The physical therapist in your hospital, along with your doctor, should supply you with a list of activities that are safe for your child to do at home. During the first few weeks it is important to prevent falls. If your child has an incision down the front of the chest, the breastbone will need special consideration. Any injury to that area, such as that of a fall, may slow the healing process of the bone. If your child is young and must be picked up, avoid lifting the child from under the arms. Instead, put one hand on the child's bottom and one behind the head. This way, you will not strain the area of the chest.

Gradually, you will be able to increase the amount of activities that your child can do. As children start to feel better, they may be more active without any encouragement. Before your child engages in any vigorous activities, such as running or sports, consult with your doctors. They should be following your child closely.

Any activity, problem, or question you may have must be directed to your physicians. Call them whenever you need answers to questions regarding your child's health. Do not be afraid to talk with your doctors. They are working for you, and for the health of your family.

Controlling Future Risk Factors

According to the American Heart Association, there are several factors that have been associated with heart disease in adults (see pages 141 through 143). Some of these factors we can control; some we cannot. However, there are a number of things that we must control. As a parent you already know that your child has heart disease at a young age. It is our job to help all of our children avoid the following future risk factors: smoking, high blood pressure, high cholesterol levels, lack of exercise, obesity, stress, and excessive alcohol intake.

Start early by educating all of your young children. Help them learn by example how to take care of themselves and grow into healthy adults. Teach them the importance of the risk factors that can have an effect on their health, and how to control them. You can do the following things, right now, to help them:

- encourage exercise;
- encourage healthy eating, and prepare meals low in cholesterol and saturated fats;
- help your children control their weight;
- keep your children away from smoke.

CHAPTER 15

Questions to Ask Your Doctor

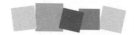

DO NOT BE AFRAID to talk to your doctors; they are human. Your doctor is not God. Chances are that your doctor is someone's husband or wife, mother or father. Doctors are people just like you. Don't be intimidated by them. In most cases, they are very dedicated professionals, who have studied hard and long to be where they are today. This makes them wealthy with information. Help them to share the wealth.

Sometimes, health professionals do not realize that the rest of the world does not always understand their "medical jargon." They will never know unless we tell them. Some doctors and nurses work every day with children who have congenital heart defects. They forget that what may be routine to them is not routine to the rest of the world, and especially not to a parent.

As parents, we have so much emotion tied up with our children and their illness. The amount of stress that we function with on a daily basis almost always affects how quickly we can understand, and how much we will remember. Sometimes, simply forming a logical sentence can be a task. Even health care professionals, doctors and nurses alike, become frantic parents when our children get sick. I believe it is human nature. Because of this, I have compiled a list of questions that you may need to ask your doctor. Write down the answers. If you do not, chances are that you will not remember the answers the next day. If any other questions arise in your mind, write them down too. They will surely escape your thoughts under stress.

Any of these questions can be modified, ignored, or expanded upon to help in your child's special circumstances. They certainly do not have to be asked in any particular order.

Questions to Ask Your Pediatric Cardiologist

1. What kind of defect does my child have?

2. Can you draw a picture of it so that I can understand better? (Use the "draw-on" picture in the back of this book.)

3. What kind of medicine will my child need?

4. Will surgery be necessary to correct the defect? If yes, how long do we have before this is necessary?

5. Do I have a choice of hospitals and surgeons? (You should always have a choice.) If yes, what are my choices, and who do you recommend? (Try: "Where would you have your child operated on, and by whom?")

Questions to Ask Your Surgeon Before Surgery

1. How long have you been performing this procedure?

2. What are the risks involved?

3. Will my child need blood transfusions?

4. Can I donate my blood to be used specifically for my child? (This is called "directed donor" blood, and every hospital should have this option. Be sure to ask this question at least two weeks before the surgery is scheduled. By donating blood directly to your child, you eliminate the risk of having the general population blood in the blood bank used. However, blood products such as platelets and plasma are usually not taken from the "directed donor" blood. These products are used frequently to stop excessive bleeding. If your child needs plasma or platelets, they will come from the blood bank.)

5. What will happen if we do not go through with this procedure?

6. What are my child's chances for a long, healthy life if we do go through with this procedure?

7. Will there be a scar? If yes, where will it be?

8. Will you be taking care of my child in the intensive care unit after surgery? If not, who will?

9. What doctor will answer my questions if you are not available?

10. How can I get in touch with you after the procedure?

Heart Defects in Children

Questions to Ask Your Surgeon Immediately After Surgery

1. Were there any problems?

2. Is my child stable?

3. Is the defect fixed?

4. Is there any chance that the defect will reoccur?

5. Is there any excessive bleeding?

6. Did my child need any blood or blood products?

7. What should I expect to see in the intensive care unit?

8. When can I see my child? Can I touch or hold my child?

9. Can I stay with my child all night?

Questions to Ask Before Your Child Is Discharged from the Hospital

1. What medicine does my child need to be on?

2. What is the medicine for, and what side effects should I watch for?

3. How long must my child be on this medicine?

4. When should I go back to the doctor with my child?

5. Which doctor should I see?

6. Are there any physical restrictions?

7. Should my child have regular rest periods?

8. Can my child swim, run, or play contact sports?

9. Is it dangerous for my child to be upset and crying?

10. Should my child be on any kind of special diet?

Part Four

Personalizing Your Child's Defect and Repair with the Use of Draw-On Hearts

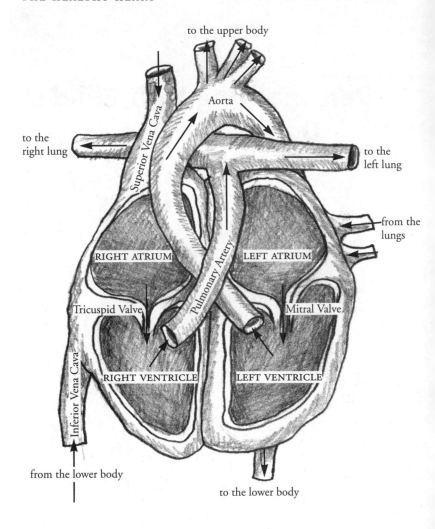

to the upper body

Aorta

Superior Vena Cava

to the
right lung

to the
left lung

from the
lungs

RIGHT ATRIUM

Pulmonary Artery

LEFT ATRIUM

Tricuspid Valve

Mitral Valve

Inferior Vena Cava

RIGHT VENTRICLE

LEFT VENTRICLE

from the lower body

to the lower body

Here is a picture of a healthy heart. You can use it to understand what has happened to your child's heart.

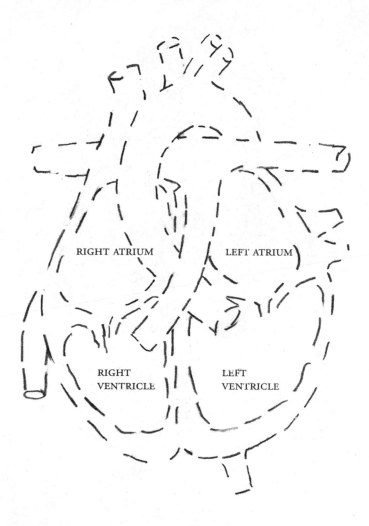

RIGHT ATRIUM

LEFT ATRIUM

RIGHT
VENTRICLE

LEFT
VENTRICLE

With a doctor's help, use this outlined heart to draw in your child's
heart defect, prior to its repair.

Date defect was diagnosed: _____

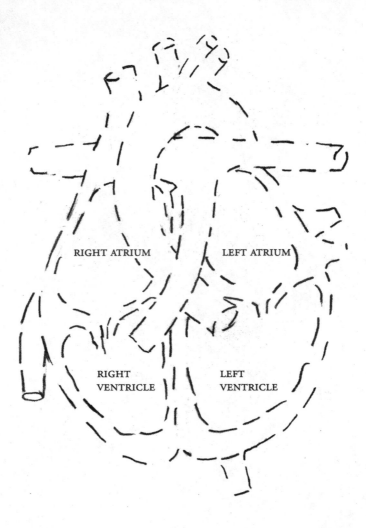

Some heart defects cannot be totally repaired with only one surgery. Use this outlined heart to draw in implanted tubes or partial corrections to your child's heart defect.

Date of partial repair: _____

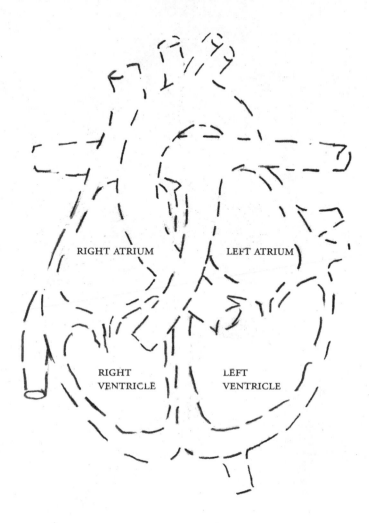

With a doctor's help, use this outlined heart to draw in the final repair of your child's heart defect.

Date of final repair: _____

Appendices

Commonly Used Medications

THE FOLLOWING IS an alphabetical list of some common medicines that you may encounter through your child's illness and recovery. This list is only a guide. Identical medicines are used every day on different children for different purposes. If your child is put on any of the following medications, speak with your physician for an accurate description of what each medicine will do for your child. Remember, no two children act and react the same way to any medical treatment. Each child may need a specific medication for a very different reason.

Because it is almost impossible to list every medicine that you will encounter, I encourage you to find a pediatric drug reference book from your local library. In general, these are some medicines that you may find. Names in parentheses are the generic trade names, not the common names.

Betadine is an antiseptic solution used to clean the skin to eliminate bacteria. It should only be used topically, never ingested.

Children's Motrin (Ibuprofen) is used mostly to decrease fevers in children but may be used for discomfort.

Codeine is a narcotic pain medication that may be used with Tylenol or cough syrup.

Coumadin (Warfarin) is a blood thinner that is taken by mouth. It is mostly used after the replacement of a heart valve. (A medication called Heparin is used for thinning the blood, too, but it is given by injection.)

Digoxin (Lanoxin) is a medication that is used to help keep the heartbeat strong and consistent.

Dobutamine is a medication that is given intravenously (IV). It is used primarily in the intensive care unit to help keep the heartbeat strong and to increase blood pressure in the body.

Dopamine is a medication that is given intravenously (IV). It is used primarily in the intensive care unit to help keep the heartbeat strong and to increase blood pressure in the body.

Heparin is a blood thinner that is given by injection or intravenously (IV). (A medication called Warfarin is also used to thin the blood, but it is given in pill form.)

Inderal (Propranolol) is a medicine used to lower the heart rate and to give the heart more time to rest. It is used to relax the muscles and vessels of the heart. It can prevent spasms and "spells" seen in children with Tetralogy of Fallot (Chapter 9).

Indocin (Indomethacin) is a medication used to decrease inflammation. It may also be used to help close a Patent Ductus Arteriosus (Chapter 5).

Lasix (Furosemide) is a diuretic; it is used to get rid of excess fluid in the body. It causes your child to urinate a lot. Lasix is often given with potassium pills because as the body excretes fluid, it also excretes electrolytes, such as potassium, which may need to be replaced.

Lidocaine is a medicine that is given intravenously (IV) to help the heart beat rhythmically and regularly.

Midazolam (Versed) is a medication that is sometimes used after surgery, or during special procedures. It helps relax the body. It will make your child very sleepy.

Morphine is a narcotic pain medicine that is often used after surgery. It is usually given intravenously (IV). Morphine may make your child very sleepy.

Nitroglycerin is used to relax the vessels in the heart. It lowers blood pressure and makes the heart's work easier.

Potassium is an electrolyte that naturally occurs in the body. It may be given as medicine to replace low blood potassium levels. Potassium is often given with Lasix, because diuretics such as Lasix tend to decrease blood potassium levels.

Pronestyl (Procanimide) is a medicine that is used to help the heart beat regularly and rhythmically.

Valium is a medicine that is sometimes used before surgery or special procedures. It helps relax the body.

Verapamil is a medicine that is sometimes used to slow down a very fast heartbeat.

Future Risk Factors

ACCORDING TO THE American Heart Association, there are several factors that have been associated with the development of heart disease in adults. By heart disease, I mean any of the following conditions:

1. high blood pressure that requires medication to control;
2. coronary artery disease, which may or may not cause angina (pain in the heart);
3. hardening or plaques in the arteries, which may cause strokes or heart attacks;
4. heart valve incompetence, even those that may have been congenital or caused by a childhood illness.

Some of the risk factors that may lead us to develop heart disease as an adult we can control. The following short list demonstrates those that we cannot control:

OUR AGE Older adults are at a higher risk of developing heart disease.

OUR SEX Men are historically more prone to heart disease than women.

OUR GENETIC MAKEUP Those of us with a strong family history of heart disease are more likely to acquire it. Strong family history in this case means that we have two or more immediate family members who have been affected with heart disease.

OUR RACE Black Americans are historically more prone to high blood pressure (which may cause heart attacks or strokes) than white Americans.

There are, however, a number of risk factors that we can control. As parents, you already know that your child has heart disease at a young age. It is our job to help all of our children avoid the following future risk factors:

SMOKING Do not expose your children to cigarette smoking. Encourage your children not to smoke by setting an example. Smoking causes the tiny arteries that supply blood flow to our hearts to constrict and go into spasm. When this happens, the heart muscle is deprived of oxygen. Cigarette smoking is dangerous to our heart's health. Please don't smoke.

HIGH BLOOD PRESSURE High blood pressure is a major contributor to heart attack and strokes. If we are overweight, our blood pressure tends to run higher. There are ways to control blood pressure through exercise and diet, but if your pressure is high, be under the care of a physician who will be able to prescribe the best possible treatment of your blood pressure. Never ignore high blood pressure.

HIGH CHOLESTEROL LEVELS High cholesterol levels in the body can cause a buildup of plaques on the walls of the arteries. These plaques can cause narrowing of the tiny arteries that bring blood to the heart muscle. Your doctor can test your blood cholesterol levels and advise you how to keep these levels under control. If your levels are too high, your doctor may prescribe medication to help bring the levels down, but this medication is rarely effective in curing high cholesterol unless we make dietary restrictions. Some foods that are high in cholesterol and saturated fat are:
a. egg yolks;
b. cream;
c. prime rib;
d. butter;
e. liver;
f. sausage;
g. whole milk hard cheeses;
h. sweet breads.

LACK OF EXERCISE A sedentary lifestyle in itself is not directly linked to heart disease, but it tends to be contributory to weight gain and overeating, which may lead to other risk factors.

OBESITY Eating too much and exercising too little may contribute to your being overweight. This places a heavy burden on your heart. It helps cause high blood pressure and can also cause some forms of diabetes, which puts an added strain on your heart. To reduce weight, see your doctor for an exercise program that is combined with a low-calorie diet.

As your children grow, keep them active and help prevent sedentary lifestyle habits, which may lead to obesity and high blood pressure. Monitor their eating habits and teach them to avoid excessive intake of foods that are very high in cholesterol and saturated fats.

STRESS Every one of us reacts differently to stress. Sometimes stress can cause us to be so upset that our blood pressure rises. Learning how to effectively cope with the daily stressors in our lives may keep us healthier. Meditation is a nice way to combat our response to a stressful life.

Help your children to verbalize feelings and cope with daily stressors, and this will help to keep them heart healthy.

Support Groups

Local Support Groups
Contact your local hospital for a list of support groups in your area. You will be relieved to know that you are not alone in dealing with a serious illness of a child. Many families have undergone events similar to your own, and you may find them an excellent source of strength.

American Heart Association
Your local chapter of the American Heart Association can be found in the White Pages of your county phone book, and can be reached via the Internet at www.AmericanHeart.org. You can also call them at 1-800/AHA-USA1.

American Academy of Pediatrics
The American Academy of Pediatrics is an organization that may be able to supply you with information on support groups in your area. They can also be reached via the Internet at www.kidsdocs@aap.org.

References

Braunwald, E., Isselbacher, K., Petersdorf, R., Wilson, Martin, D., Fauci, M. 1987. *Harrison's Principles of Internal Medicine.* 11th ed. New York: McGraw-Hill.

Cataldo, Whinney. 1983. *Understanding Normal and Clinical Nutrition.* St. Paul: West.

Fyler, Donald C. 1992. *Nadas' Pediatric Cardiology.* Philadelphia: Hanley and Belfus.

Hole, John W., Jr. 1984. *Human Anatomy and Physiology.* 3rd ed. Dubuque, IA: Wm. C. Brown.

Jacobs, Marshall L., and Norwood, William I. 1992. *Pediatric Cardiac Anesthesia.* Stoneham, MA: Butterworth-Heinemann.

Kirklin, John W., and Barratt-Boyes, Brian G. 1993. *Cardiac Surgery.* 2d ed. New York: Churchill Livingstone.

Mavroudis, Constantine, and Backer, Carl L. 1994. *Pediatric Cardiac Surgery.* 2d ed. St. Louis: Mosby.

Milunsky, A., ed. 1986. *Genetic Disorders of the Fetus: Diagnosis, Prevention, and Treatment.* 2d ed. New York: Plenum.

Pongpanich, B., Sueblinvong, V., and Vongprateep C., eds. 1990. *Pediatric Cardiology.* Amsterdam: Elsevier.

Urdang, Laurence, and Swallow, Helen Harding, eds. 1983. *Mosby's Medical and Nursing Dictionary.* St. Louis: C. V. Mosby.

Index

Heart Defects in Children

Heart Defects in Children